The Complete MCAS Guide

Managing Mast Cell Activation Syndrome from Diagnosis to Long-Term Wellness

Stella Marion Kaufman

number) immediately. Do not rely on information in this book for emergency medical situations.

Individual Results Disclaimer: The strategies and information presented in this book may not be suitable for every individual. Results and experiences may vary significantly between individuals based on their unique medical history, current health status, genetic factors, and other variables.

Case Study Disclaimer: The names and scenarios depicted in this book are purely for illustrative purposes only. Any resemblance to actual persons, living or dead, or actual events is purely coincidental. Case examples are composites created for educational purposes and do not represent specific individuals.

Research Disclaimer: While this book references current research and medical literature, the field of mast cell disorders continues to evolve rapidly. New research may supersede or modify the information presented herein.

Liability Disclaimer: The author and publisher disclaim any liability for any adverse effects or consequences resulting from the use of any information, suggestions, or procedures described in this book. Readers assume full responsibility for consulting with appropriate medical professionals regarding their health and medical decisions.

By reading and using this book, you acknowledge that you have read and understood this disclaimer and agree to its terms.

ISBN: 978-1-7641438-4-4

Isohan Publishing

Table of Contents

Chapter 1: MCAS Fundamentals

Your Mast Cells and What Goes Wrong

Your body contains an intricate network of cellular defenders, each with specific roles in keeping you healthy and protected. Among these defenders are mast cells - specialized immune cells that most people never think about until something goes wrong. Think of mast cells as your body's security guards, stationed throughout your tissues, ready to respond when they detect a threat. But what happens when these security guards become overly sensitive, responding to everyday situations as if they were life-threatening emergencies?

What Are Mast Cells - The Body's Sentinel Guards

Mast cells are ancient protectors that have been part of human biology for millions of years. These cells originated as our first line of defense against parasites and infections, particularly those that could breach our skin and mucosal barriers. Dr. Paul Ehrlich first discovered them in 1878, naming them "Mastzellen" because they appeared to be well-fed cells packed with granules.

These remarkable cells position themselves strategically throughout your body - in your skin, lungs, digestive tract, blood vessels, and nervous system. They're particularly concentrated at the interfaces between your body and the outside world: your skin, respiratory tract, and gastrointestinal system. This positioning makes perfect sense when you consider their role as sentinel guards, watching for potential threats that might enter your body through these pathways (1).

Inside each mast cell are hundreds of tiny storage compartments called granules, packed with over 200 different chemical mediators. The most famous of these is histamine, but mast cells also store tryptase, heparin, cytokines, leukotrienes, and prostaglandins. When a mast cell detects a threat, it can release these mediators within seconds - a process called degranulation. This rapid response system allowed our ancestors to survive encounters with dangerous parasites and toxins (2).

Consider Sarah, a 34-year-old teacher who first learned about mast cells after years of mysterious symptoms. "I never knew these cells existed until my doctor explained why I was reacting to everything," she recalls. "Once I understood that my mast cells were trying to protect me but were overreacting, it completely changed how I viewed my symptoms. Instead of feeling like my body was betraying me, I realized it was working too hard to keep me safe."

Normal vs. Abnormal Mast Cell Activation

Under normal circumstances, mast cells maintain a careful balance. They respond appropriately to genuine threats while remaining calm in the face of harmless substances. This balance depends on complex signaling pathways that tell the cell when to activate and when to remain quiet.

Normal mast cell activation occurs when you encounter actual threats - certain bacteria, viruses, or parasites. The cells release just enough mediators to eliminate the threat and then return to their resting state. This response is localized, proportionate, and temporary. For example, when you get a small cut, mast cells in the area release histamine to increase blood flow and bring immune cells to the site.

You might notice some redness and swelling, but the response resolves as the wound heals.

In MCAS, this carefully orchestrated system goes awry. Mast cells become hyperreactive, responding to normal, everyday triggers as if they were dangerous threats. They may release excessive amounts of mediators, release them for prolonged periods, or respond to substances that shouldn't trigger them at all. This abnormal activation can occur spontaneously or in response to triggers that most people tolerate without issue (3).

The triggers that can activate mast cells in MCAS are surprisingly diverse. They include:

Physical triggers: Heat, cold, pressure, vibration, exercise, and sunlight can all cause mast cell activation in sensitive individuals. Maria, a 28-year-old nurse, discovered that even the friction from her work scrubs could trigger a reaction. "I thought I was developing allergies to my uniform material, but it turned out to be the physical pressure and friction causing my mast cells to react."

Chemical triggers: Fragrances, cleaning products, medications, food additives, and environmental chemicals can trigger reactions. These aren't true allergic responses but rather direct mast cell activation. Tom, a 45-year-old accountant, found that walking through the cleaning supply aisle at the grocery store would leave him feeling dizzy and nauseous for hours.

Emotional and physical stress: The nervous system and immune system communicate closely, and stress can directly trigger mast cell activation. This connection explains why symptoms often worsen during stressful periods or why some people experience reactions during emotional situations.

Hormonal changes: Many people with MCAS notice that their symptoms fluctuate with hormonal cycles, pregnancy, or menopause. The connection between hormones and mast cells helps explain why MCAS symptoms often change throughout a person's life.

The Inflammatory Cascade - From Trigger to Symptom

Understanding how a trigger becomes a symptom helps you recognize and manage your reactions more effectively. The process begins when a trigger encounters a mast cell, either directly or through other immune cells that signal the mast cell to activate.

The first phase happens within seconds to minutes. The mast cell rapidly releases preformed mediators stored in its granules. Histamine causes blood vessels to dilate and become leaky, leading to swelling, redness, and increased mucus production. Tryptase, another major mediator, can be measured in blood tests and serves as a biomarker for mast cell activation. Heparin affects blood clotting, while various cytokines signal other immune cells to join the response (4).

The second phase occurs over minutes to hours as the mast cell manufactures new mediators. Leukotrienes cause prolonged inflammation and bronchoconstriction. Prostaglandins contribute to pain, fever, and cardiovascular effects. This phase explains why some reactions seem to have two waves - an immediate response followed by a delayed, sometimes more severe reaction.

The symptoms you experience depend on where the mast cells are activated and which mediators they release.

Activation in the skin causes hives, flushing, or itching. Activation in the respiratory tract leads to congestion, coughing, or difficulty breathing. Gastrointestinal activation results in nausea, cramping, or diarrhea. Cardiovascular activation can cause rapid heart rate, blood pressure changes, or even fainting.

Jennifer, a 41-year-old mother of two, describes her typical reaction: "It usually starts with a feeling of warmth and flushing in my face and chest. Within about ten minutes, my heart starts racing, and I feel nauseous. If it's a bad reaction, I'll get stomach cramps and have to use the bathroom urgently. The whole thing can last anywhere from thirty minutes to several hours, depending on what triggered it."

MCAS vs. Mastocytosis vs. Hereditary Alpha Tryptasemia

Many people receive their MCAS diagnosis after being evaluated for other mast cell disorders. Understanding the distinctions between these conditions helps clarify why your symptoms occur and what treatment approaches might work best.

Mastocytosis involves an abnormal accumulation of mast cells in tissues. In this condition, there are simply too many mast cells present, and they may also behave abnormally. Mastocytosis can be diagnosed through skin biopsies or bone marrow biopsies that show increased numbers of mast cells. The condition often presents with characteristic skin lesions called urticaria pigmentosa, though not all patients develop these lesions (5).

MCAS, in contrast, involves normal numbers of mast cells that behave abnormally. The cells are hyperreactive and release excessive mediators in response to inappropriate triggers. Diagnosis relies on clinical symptoms, evidence of mast cell activation (such as elevated tryptase during reactions), and response to mast cell-targeted treatments.

Hereditary Alpha Tryptasemia (HαT) is a recently recognized genetic condition that involves elevated baseline tryptase levels due to extra copies of the alpha tryptase gene. People with HαT may experience some MCAS-like symptoms, but the condition has distinct features and may require different management approaches (6).

Dr. Michael, an allergist specializing in mast cell disorders, explains: "I often see patients who have been told they have allergies, anxiety, or irritable bowel syndrome before receiving an MCAS diagnosis. The key is recognizing that these symptoms can all stem from mast cell activation and that treating the underlying mast cell dysfunction can provide relief across multiple body systems."

The Multi-System Nature of MCAS

One of the most challenging aspects of MCAS is its ability to affect virtually every organ system in your body. This occurs because mast cells are distributed throughout your tissues and release mediators that have wide-ranging effects. Understanding this multi-system nature helps explain why MCAS symptoms can seem so diverse and unrelated.

Dermatologic symptoms are among the most common and visible manifestations of MCAS. Flushing, hives, itching, and skin sensitivity can occur anywhere on the body. Some people develop chronic conditions like eczema or experience unusual reactions to skincare products, soaps, or clothing materials.

Gastrointestinal symptoms affect the majority of MCAS patients. These can include nausea, vomiting, abdominal pain, cramping, diarrhea, constipation, and food sensitivities. The digestive tract contains large numbers of mast cells, particularly in areas like the stomach and small intestine, making it a common site for reactions.

Respiratory symptoms range from nasal congestion and post-nasal drip to coughing, wheezing, and shortness of breath. Some people experience a sensation of throat tightness or feel like they can't get enough air, even when their oxygen levels are normal.

Cardiovascular symptoms can be particularly frightening and include rapid heart rate, blood pressure fluctuations, chest pain, and episodes of fainting or near-fainting. These symptoms occur because mast cell mediators directly affect blood vessels and heart function.

Neurological symptoms may include brain fog, difficulty concentrating, headaches, dizziness, and mood changes. The blood-brain barrier contains mast cells, and activation in the nervous system can affect cognitive function and emotional stability.

Genitourinary symptoms can include frequent urination, pelvic pain, and in women, menstrual irregularities or painful periods. The relationship between hormones and mast cells means that symptoms often fluctuate with the menstrual cycle.

Lisa, a 39-year-old graphic designer, describes living with multi-system MCAS: "Before my diagnosis, I felt like I was falling apart. I had skin problems, stomach issues, heart palpitations, and brain fog. Different doctors wanted to treat each symptom separately, but nothing worked long-term. Once I understood that all these symptoms were connected through mast cell activation, I could finally start addressing the root cause instead of just managing individual symptoms."

Moving Forward with Understanding

Understanding the fundamentals of MCAS provides the foundation for everything that follows in your journey toward better health. These cellular security guards that have protected humans for millennia are simply doing their job too enthusiastically in your body. This knowledge transforms your relationship with your symptoms from fear and confusion to understanding and empowerment.

Your mast cells aren't betraying you - they're protecting you with outdated information about what constitutes a threat. With proper management, you can help retrain them to respond more appropriately while avoiding the triggers that send them into overdrive.

The path forward involves learning to work with your mast cells rather than against them, understanding your personal patterns of activation, and developing strategies to maintain stability while living fully. This foundation of understanding makes every subsequent step in your MCAS management more effective and meaningful.

Key Learning Points

- Mast cells are immune system guards positioned throughout your body to detect and respond to threats

- MCAS occurs when these normally protective cells become overreactive to everyday triggers

- Symptoms can affect multiple body systems because mast cells are distributed widely throughout your tissues

- The condition involves normal numbers of mast cells behaving abnormally, distinguishing it from mastocytosis

- Understanding your body's protective mechanisms helps transform fear into informed action

- Multi-system symptoms that seem unrelated often share the common thread of mast cell activation

Chapter 2: The Diagnostic Journey

Walking into yet another doctor's office with a list of seemingly unrelated symptoms can feel like preparing for battle. You've learned to expect the skeptical glances, the suggestions that stress might be the culprit, or the recommendations for anxiety medication when what you really need are answers. The diagnostic journey for MCAS often spans years and multiple healthcare providers before you finally find someone who understands what you're experiencing.

This process isn't just about getting a diagnosis - it's about finding validation for your symptoms, understanding what's happening in your body, and building a healthcare team that can support your long-term wellness. While the journey can be frustrating, understanding what to expect and how to prepare can make the process more manageable and successful.

The Challenge of MCAS Diagnosis

MCAS diagnosis presents unique challenges that stem from both the nature of the condition and the current state of medical education. Most healthcare providers receive minimal training about mast cell disorders during their medical education, and MCAS has only been formally recognized as a distinct condition since the early 2000s. This means that many doctors are still learning about the condition alongside their patients (7).

The symptoms of MCAS often mimic other conditions, leading to a phenomenon known as diagnostic overshadowing. Dr. Jennifer, an internal medicine physician who developed MCAS herself, explains: "Before I understood

MCAS, I probably diagnosed dozens of patients with irritable bowel syndrome, anxiety disorders, or fibromyalgia who actually had mast cell activation. The symptoms are real and significant, but without understanding the underlying mechanism, we treat each symptom separately instead of addressing the root cause."

The intermittent nature of MCAS symptoms adds another layer of complexity. Unlike conditions with constant, predictable symptoms, MCAS can cause periods of relative wellness followed by sudden, severe reactions. You might feel completely normal during your doctor's appointment, making it difficult to convey the severity of your symptoms during flares.

Traditional diagnostic approaches in medicine rely heavily on objective findings - abnormal blood tests, imaging results, or physical examination findings. MCAS diagnosis, however, often depends on clinical presentation and response to treatment, which can make some healthcare providers uncomfortable. The condition requires doctors to listen carefully to patient narratives and consider patterns of symptoms over time.

Mark, a 52-year-old engineer, spent five years seeking a diagnosis: "I saw twelve different doctors before finding one who understood MCAS. Each specialist focused on their area - the cardiologist looked at my heart palpitations, the gastroenterologist treated my digestive issues, the dermatologist prescribed creams for my skin problems. No one stepped back to see the bigger picture until I found a physician familiar with mast cell disorders."

Diagnostic Criteria and Biomarkers

The diagnosis of MCAS relies on established criteria that help differentiate the condition from other disorders. Understanding these criteria helps you work more effectively with your healthcare providers and ensures that appropriate testing is performed.

The current diagnostic criteria for MCAS include three main components: clinical symptoms consistent with mast cell activation, evidence of mast cell activation through laboratory testing, and response to medications that target mast cell mediators or block their effects (8).

Clinical symptoms must involve at least two organ systems and be consistent with mast cell mediator release. The symptoms should be episodic and recurrent, often triggered by identifiable factors. Healthcare providers look for patterns that suggest mast cell activation rather than other disease processes.

Laboratory evidence of mast cell activation can be challenging to obtain because it often requires testing during or immediately after a reaction. The most commonly used biomarker is serum tryptase, which should be measured during a reaction and compared to baseline levels. An elevation of 20% plus 2 ng/mL above baseline is considered significant. However, tryptase elevations don't occur in all patients or with all reactions, so normal levels don't rule out MCAS (9).

Other laboratory markers that may support the diagnosis include elevated histamine or histamine metabolites in urine, elevated prostaglandin D2 or its metabolite in urine, and elevated leukotrienes. These tests are often more difficult to obtain and interpret than tryptase levels.

Response to treatment with mast cell-directed therapies provides additional support for the diagnosis. Patients with MCAS typically experience improvement when treated with antihistamines, mast cell stabilizers, or other medications that target mast cell mediators. This therapeutic response can be as important as laboratory findings in confirming the diagnosis.

Dr. Sarah, an allergist specializing in MCAS, notes: "I often tell patients that MCAS diagnosis is like putting together a puzzle. We look at the clinical picture, any laboratory evidence we can obtain, and how you respond to treatment. Sometimes the response to treatment is the most convincing piece of evidence we have."

The challenge with laboratory testing lies in timing and availability. Many reactions occur unpredictably, making it difficult to obtain blood or urine samples during the acute phase. Some patients need to be taught how to recognize the early signs of a reaction so they can seek immediate testing.

Rachel, a 33-year-old accountant, describes her testing experience: "My doctor gave me lab slips to carry with me and instructions to go to the emergency department or urgent care for blood work if I had a severe reaction. It took three episodes before we caught one with elevated tryptase levels, but having that objective evidence made all the difference in getting other providers to take my symptoms seriously."

Essential Tests and When to Order Them

Understanding which tests are most useful for MCAS diagnosis and when to order them helps you advocate for appropriate evaluation. The timing and interpretation of these tests require coordination between you and your healthcare provider.

Baseline tryptase should be measured when you're feeling well and haven't had a recent reaction. This establishes your normal level, which is essential for interpreting acute measurements. Some people have naturally elevated baseline tryptase levels, which may suggest Hereditary Alpha Tryptasemia or other conditions.

Acute tryptase should be measured during or within 1-4 hours of a significant reaction. The timing is critical because tryptase levels peak quickly and then decline. This test is most likely to be positive with severe, systemic reactions rather than mild, localized symptoms.

24-hour urine studies can measure histamine and its metabolites (N-methylhistamine), prostaglandin D2 metabolites, or leukotriene metabolites. These tests can sometimes detect mast cell activation even when tryptase levels remain normal. The collection process requires careful attention to timing and storage requirements.

Additional blood tests might include complete blood counts to look for eosinophilia or other abnormalities, vitamin B12 and folate levels (which can be elevated in mast cell disorders), and serum immunoglobulin E levels.

Genetic testing for Hereditary Alpha Tryptasemia may be recommended if you have persistently elevated baseline tryptase levels or a family history suggestive of mast cell disorders.

The decision about which tests to order and when depends on your specific symptoms, the availability of testing during reactions, and your healthcare provider's experience with MCAS. Some tests are expensive or not covered by insurance, so prioritizing the most likely to be helpful is important.

Dr. Michael explains his approach: "I usually start with baseline tryptase and a 24-hour urine study for histamine metabolites because these can be done at any time. If those are normal but the clinical picture strongly suggests MCAS, I might recommend more specialized testing or consider a therapeutic trial of mast cell-directed medications."

Finding the Right Specialists

The search for healthcare providers who understand MCAS can be one of the most challenging aspects of your diagnostic journey. While awareness of the condition is growing, many areas still lack specialists familiar with mast cell disorders.

Allergists and immunologists are often the most knowledgeable about MCAS, particularly those who specialize in complex allergic conditions or have specific interest in mast cell disorders. However, not all allergists are familiar with MCAS, so research their background and ask about their experience with mast cell conditions.

Hematologists may be involved in your care, particularly if mastocytosis needs to be ruled out. These specialists are familiar with blood disorders and can perform bone marrow biopsies if needed.

Gastroenterologists might be helpful if your primary symptoms involve the digestive system, though they need to be open to considering MCAS rather than focusing solely on traditional gastrointestinal disorders.

Primary care providers who are willing to learn about MCAS can become valuable members of your healthcare team. Some family physicians and internists have educated themselves about mast cell disorders and can provide excellent ongoing care.

Finding specialists often requires detective work. Online support groups, patient advocacy organizations, and physician referral networks can provide recommendations. The International Chronic Urticaria Society and The Mastocytosis Society maintain lists of healthcare providers with expertise in mast cell conditions.

When evaluating potential providers, consider asking about their experience with MCAS, their familiarity with current diagnostic criteria, and their approach to treatment. Providers who are willing to collaborate with you and consider your symptom patterns are more likely to provide effective care than those who dismiss symptoms they can't immediately explain.

Janet, a 44-year-old teacher, describes finding her specialist: "I drove four hours to see an allergist who was recommended by another MCAS patient. During our first appointment, she spent ninety minutes listening to my history and didn't once suggest that my symptoms were anxiety-related. She understood the connection between all my different symptoms and had a clear plan for testing and treatment. The drive was worth it to finally feel heard and understood."

Preparing for Medical Appointments

Effective preparation for medical appointments can make the difference between a frustrating encounter and a productive step forward in your diagnosis. Healthcare providers often have limited time, so presenting your information clearly and concisely helps them understand your situation quickly.

Symptom documentation should include detailed records of your symptoms, their timing, potential triggers, and severity. Many patients find it helpful to use symptom tracking apps or maintain written logs. Include photographs of visible symptoms like rashes or swelling when possible.

Trigger identification helps providers understand patterns in your symptoms. Keep records of foods, activities, environmental exposures, stressors, or other factors that seem to precede reactions. Even if you're not certain about triggers, documenting correlations can provide valuable information.

Medical history organization should include previous diagnoses, treatments tried, medications (including dosages and responses), and any relevant family history. Bringing copies of previous test results saves time and prevents unnecessary repeat testing.

Current symptom assessment before each appointment helps you accurately describe your recent status. Many people with MCAS experience good days and bad days, so having a clear picture of your recent symptom pattern helps providers understand your current state.

Question preparation ensures you address your most important concerns during the appointment. Write down questions in advance and prioritize them, starting with the most pressing issues.

Support person can be valuable during appointments, particularly for complex discussions about diagnosis and treatment. A friend or family member can help remember important information and provide emotional support during potentially stressful medical encounters.

Dr. Lisa, a family physician experienced with MCAS, offers this advice: "Patients who come prepared with organized information help me provide better care. When someone can clearly describe their symptom patterns and potential triggers, I can focus on interpretation and treatment planning rather than spending most of our time gathering basic information."

Working with Insurance and Medical Records

Insurance coverage for MCAS-related care can be challenging because the condition is still relatively unknown to many insurance reviewers. Understanding how to work within insurance systems helps ensure you receive needed care while minimizing financial burden.

Pre-authorization may be required for specialized testing, particularly expensive tests like genetic studies or specialized urine studies. Work with your healthcare provider's office to submit appropriate documentation supporting the medical necessity of requested tests.

Documentation of medical necessity should clearly link requested tests or treatments to your symptoms and potential MCAS diagnosis. Healthcare providers experienced with MCAS understand how to write justifications that insurance companies are more likely to approve.

Appeal processes may be necessary if initial requests are denied. Many denials are overturned on appeal, particularly when additional medical documentation is provided. Patient advocacy organizations can sometimes provide guidance on effective appeal strategies.

Medical records management becomes increasingly important as you see multiple providers and undergo various tests. Keeping your own copies of test results, consultation notes, and treatment records ensures continuity of care and prevents loss of important information.

The diagnostic journey for MCAS requires persistence, organization, and often significant personal advocacy. While the process can be lengthy and sometimes frustrating, understanding what to expect and how to prepare increases your chances of obtaining an accurate diagnosis and effective treatment plan.

Building relationships with knowledgeable healthcare providers, maintaining detailed symptom records, and staying informed about current MCAS research and treatment approaches will serve you well throughout your ongoing care. The investment in obtaining an accurate diagnosis pays dividends in improved symptom management and quality of life.

Charting Your Path to Answers

The diagnostic journey for MCAS represents more than simply obtaining a medical label for your symptoms. It marks the beginning of understanding your body's unique patterns and building the foundation for effective long-term management. While the path to diagnosis can test your patience and persistence, each step forward brings you closer to the relief and validation you deserve.

Your role as an active participant in this process cannot be overstated. The detailed observations you make about your symptoms, triggers, and responses to treatments provide invaluable information that guides your healthcare team's decisions. Your persistence in seeking answers, even when faced with skepticism or dismissal, ultimately leads to better care not just for yourself but for future patients who will benefit from increased awareness of MCAS.

The relationships you build with knowledgeable healthcare providers become the cornerstone of your ongoing wellness strategy. These partnerships, built on mutual respect and shared understanding of your condition, will serve you well beyond the initial diagnosis as you work together to optimize your treatment and maintain your health over time.

Key Learning Points

- MCAS diagnosis requires clinical symptoms, laboratory evidence, and treatment response rather than a single definitive test

- Finding knowledgeable healthcare providers often requires research and persistence, but the effort is worthwhile

- Detailed symptom documentation and trigger identification significantly improve diagnostic accuracy

- Laboratory testing timing is critical, with some tests requiring collection during active reactions

- Insurance navigation requires understanding medical necessity documentation and appeal processes

- Building strong provider relationships creates the foundation for long-term successful management

Chapter 3: MCAS Phenotypes and Presentations

- Recognizing Your Unique MCAS Pattern

Every person with MCAS experiences the condition differently, creating a unique fingerprint of symptoms, triggers, and responses that can vary dramatically from one individual to another. Understanding that MCAS isn't a one-size-fits-all condition helps explain why your experience might differ significantly from others with the same diagnosis and why treatment approaches that work for some people may not work for you.

This variation isn't a flaw in the diagnostic process or a sign that your symptoms aren't real. Instead, it reflects the complex nature of mast cell biology and the individual factors that influence how your particular mast cells respond to triggers. Recognizing your personal MCAS phenotype - your unique pattern of symptoms and triggers - becomes the foundation for developing an effective, personalized management strategy.

The Spectrum of MCAS Presentations

MCAS exists on a spectrum from mild, intermittent symptoms that cause occasional inconvenience to severe, life-threatening reactions that significantly impact daily functioning. This spectrum reflects differences in the number of mast cells activated, the mediators they release, the tissues where activation occurs, and individual sensitivity to these mediators.

Some people experience what might be called "mild MCAS," with symptoms that are manageable and don't significantly interfere with daily activities. These individuals might have occasional digestive upset after eating certain foods, mild skin reactions to fragrances, or periodic episodes of fatigue and brain fog. While these symptoms are real and can be frustrating, they don't typically require emergency care or cause major lifestyle modifications.

At the other end of the spectrum are individuals with severe MCAS who experience frequent, intense reactions that can be life-threatening. These people might have multiple severe food and environmental sensitivities, require emergency care for reactions, and need to make significant lifestyle modifications to maintain stability. Between these extremes lies the majority of MCAS patients, who experience moderate symptoms that wax and wane over time.

Dr. Patricia, an immunologist specializing in mast cell disorders, observes: "I see patients across the entire spectrum of MCAS severity. What's important to understand is that mild symptoms can become severe if not properly managed, and severe symptoms can often be brought under better control with appropriate treatment. The key is recognizing where you fall on this spectrum and developing management strategies that match your needs."

The factors that influence where someone falls on this spectrum include genetic predisposition, environmental exposures, concurrent health conditions, stress levels, hormonal status, and the effectiveness of treatment interventions. These factors can change over time, meaning that your MCAS presentation might evolve throughout your life.

Understanding your position on this spectrum helps set realistic expectations for treatment outcomes and helps you communicate effectively with healthcare providers about the impact of your symptoms. It also helps you connect with other patients who have similar experiences and can offer relevant advice and support.

Gastrointestinal-Dominant MCAS

For many people with MCAS, the digestive system bears the brunt of mast cell activation. The gastrointestinal tract contains large numbers of mast cells, particularly in the stomach, small intestine, and colon, making it a common site for symptoms. Gastrointestinal-dominant MCAS can significantly impact nutrition, social activities, and quality of life.

The symptoms of GI-dominant MCAS often begin subtly and may be initially attributed to common digestive disorders. Patients frequently receive diagnoses of irritable bowel syndrome, gastroesophageal reflux disease, or functional dyspepsia before the underlying mast cell activation is recognized. The key difference is that MCAS-related GI symptoms often occur in response to specific triggers and may be accompanied by symptoms in other body systems.

Stomach symptoms commonly include nausea, bloating, early satiety (feeling full quickly), and epigastric pain. Some people experience gastroparesis-like symptoms, where the stomach empties slowly, leading to prolonged feelings of fullness and discomfort. Acid production may be affected, leading to either excessive acid and heartburn or insufficient acid and poor digestion.

Small intestine symptoms often involve cramping, diarrhea, and malabsorption. The rapid transit time associated with mast cell activation can prevent proper nutrient absorption, leading to deficiencies in vitamins and minerals. Some patients develop signs of small intestinal bacterial overgrowth (SIBO) as a secondary complication.

Large intestine symptoms include urgency, frequent bowel movements, mucus production, and abdominal cramping. The inflammation caused by mast cell activation can affect the normal bacterial balance in the colon and interfere with water absorption.

Maria, a 31-year-old marketing professional, describes her GI-dominant MCAS: "For years, I thought I just had a 'sensitive stomach.' I couldn't eat out without worrying about getting sick, and I was constantly dealing with nausea and stomach cramps. I tried every diet and elimination protocol you can imagine. It wasn't until I connected my digestive symptoms with my skin reactions and realized they often occurred together that my doctor started investigating MCAS."

The triggers for GI-dominant MCAS extend beyond just food sensitivities. While certain foods (particularly high-histamine foods, food additives, and individual trigger foods) commonly cause symptoms, other factors can also activate intestinal mast cells. Stress, infections, medications, and even changes in weather can trigger GI symptoms in sensitive individuals.

Managing GI-dominant MCAS often requires a multi-faceted approach that addresses both the underlying mast cell activation and the secondary effects on digestive function. This might include dietary modifications, medications to stabilize mast cells, treatments for associated conditions like SIBO, and supplements to address nutritional deficiencies.

The social impact of GI-dominant MCAS can be significant. Many patients report feeling anxious about eating in restaurants, traveling, or attending social events where food is involved. The unpredictable nature of symptoms can make it difficult to plan activities and can strain relationships with family and friends who may not understand the severity of the condition.

Cardiovascular-Dominant MCAS

Mast cells are found throughout the cardiovascular system, including the heart muscle, blood vessel walls, and surrounding tissues. When these cells activate, they can cause a range of cardiovascular symptoms that can be frightening and sometimes dangerous. Cardiovascular-dominant MCAS often leads patients to emergency departments and cardiology consultations before the underlying mast cell activation is recognized.

Heart rate abnormalities are among the most common cardiovascular manifestations of MCAS. Patients may experience rapid heart rate (tachycardia), irregular rhythms, or a sensation that their heart is pounding or racing. These symptoms can occur at rest or be triggered by minimal exertion, eating, or exposure to triggers.

Blood pressure fluctuations can include both high and low blood pressure episodes. Some patients experience sudden drops in blood pressure that can cause dizziness, fainting, or near-fainting episodes. Others may have episodes of elevated blood pressure during reactions. The variability in blood pressure can make it challenging to manage with conventional medications.

Chest symptoms may include chest pain, pressure, or tightness. These symptoms can mimic heart attack symptoms, leading to multiple emergency department visits and extensive cardiac workups that often return normal results. The chest discomfort in MCAS is typically related to inflammation and blood vessel changes rather than blocked coronary arteries.

Flushing and temperature regulation problems occur when mast cells in blood vessels release mediators that cause vasodilation. This can lead to episodes of flushing, feeling overheated, or difficulty regulating body temperature. Some patients experience these symptoms as waves of heat that can be quite uncomfortable.

James, a 48-year-old construction manager, experienced cardiovascular-dominant MCAS: "I ended up in the emergency room six times in one year because of chest pain and heart palpitations. Every time, they did EKGs, blood tests, and even a stress test, but everything was normal. The cardiologist kept telling me it was anxiety, but I knew something physical was happening. It wasn't until an allergist measured my tryptase during one of these episodes that we discovered it was mast cell activation affecting my heart."

The triggers for cardiovascular symptoms in MCAS can be diverse and sometimes unexpected. Physical exertion, heat exposure, emotional stress, certain foods, medications, and even changes in posture can trigger cardiovascular reactions. Some patients develop a condition called postural orthostatic tachycardia syndrome (POTS) as a secondary complication of MCAS.

Diagnosis of cardiovascular-dominant MCAS often requires ruling out primary cardiac conditions while documenting the relationship between symptoms and mast cell activation. This may involve wearing heart monitors during symptomatic periods, measuring tryptase levels during cardiovascular episodes, and demonstrating improvement with mast cell-directed treatments.

Treatment typically involves medications that stabilize mast cells, manage specific cardiovascular symptoms, and avoid known triggers. Some patients benefit from medications commonly used for POTS, such as fludrocortisone or beta-blockers, in addition to mast cell-specific treatments.

Neurological-Dominant MCAS

The nervous system's relationship with mast cells is particularly complex, with mast cells found throughout the brain, spinal cord, and peripheral nervous system. These cells can cross the blood-brain barrier and directly affect neurological function through the release of inflammatory mediators. Neurological-dominant MCAS often presents with symptoms that can be mistaken for psychiatric conditions, neurodegenerative diseases, or other neurological disorders.

Cognitive symptoms represent some of the most challenging aspects of neurological MCAS. Brain fog - a term that encompasses difficulty concentrating, memory problems, and mental fatigue - affects the majority of patients with this presentation. The fog can range from mild difficulty finding words to severe impairment that affects work performance and daily functioning.

Mood and behavioral changes occur when mast cell mediators affect brain regions responsible for emotional regulation. Patients may experience increased anxiety, depression, irritability, or mood swings that seem disproportionate to their circumstances. These changes often correlate with other MCAS symptoms, helping to distinguish them from primary psychiatric conditions.

Headaches and migraines are common in neurological MCAS, often triggered by the same factors that cause other mast cell symptoms. The inflammation caused by mast cell activation can trigger severe headaches that may be accompanied by nausea, sensitivity to light and sound, and visual disturbances.

Sleep disturbances can include difficulty falling asleep, frequent awakening, non-restorative sleep, and vivid dreams or nightmares. The inflammatory mediators released by activated mast cells can disrupt normal sleep architecture, leading to chronic fatigue and worsening of other symptoms.

Sensory symptoms may include numbness, tingling, burning sensations, or heightened sensitivity to touch, sound, or light. Some patients experience a condition called hypervigilance, where they become extremely sensitive to environmental stimuli that most people easily ignore.

Dr. Rebecca, a neurologist who has studied MCAS extensively, explains: "What makes neurological MCAS particularly challenging is that the symptoms can be subtle and subjective. Patients often feel like they're not being taken seriously when they describe brain fog or sensitivity to stimuli. However, when we measure inflammatory markers in the cerebrospinal fluid or see improvement with mast cell treatments, it becomes clear that there's a real biological basis for these symptoms."

Amanda, a 36-year-old software engineer, describes her neurological symptoms: "The brain fog was the worst part. I went from being sharp and quick-thinking to feeling like I was trying to think through molasses. I would sit at my computer and forget what I was supposed to be working on. I thought I was developing early-onset dementia until my doctor connected it to my other MCAS symptoms and started me on mast cell stabilizers."

The triggers for neurological MCAS symptoms often overlap with those that cause systemic reactions. Stress, certain foods, environmental exposures, hormonal changes, and infections can all trigger neurological symptoms. The connection between stress and symptom worsening creates a challenging cycle where neurological symptoms increase stress, which then worsens the symptoms.

Diagnosis of neurological-dominant MCAS requires careful evaluation to rule out other neurological conditions while documenting the relationship between symptoms and mast cell activation. Neuropsychological testing may reveal patterns consistent with inflammatory brain conditions, and some patients benefit from specialized imaging studies that can detect brain inflammation.

Treatment approaches for neurological MCAS often include medications that can cross the blood-brain barrier to stabilize mast cells in the nervous system. Some patients benefit from supplements that support brain health and reduce inflammation, while others need medications specifically targeting neurological symptoms alongside their general MCAS treatments.

Skin-Dominant MCAS

The skin contains numerous mast cells, particularly in areas exposed to potential environmental threats. Skin-dominant MCAS often presents with visible symptoms that can be easier to recognize and document than internal symptoms, though they can be socially challenging and emotionally distressing for patients.

Hives and angioedema are classic manifestations of skin mast cell activation. Hives can appear anywhere on the body and may be small and localized or large and widespread. They typically itch intensely and can appear and disappear rapidly. Angioedema involves deeper swelling, particularly around the eyes, lips, and throat, and can be dangerous if it affects breathing.

Flushing and erythema occur when mast cells in blood vessels release mediators that cause vasodilation. This can create redness and warmth in affected areas, most commonly the face, neck, and chest. Some patients experience episodic flushing that comes and goes, while others have persistent redness.

Itching and burning sensations can occur even without visible skin changes. Patients may experience intense itching that seems to come from within the skin rather than on the surface. Some describe burning, stinging, or crawling sensations that can be quite distressing.

Skin sensitivity and reactivity can make it difficult to use normal skincare products, detergents, or clothing materials. The skin may react to physical stimuli like pressure, heat, cold, or friction. Some patients develop a condition called dermatographism, where writing on the skin with a blunt object creates raised, itchy marks.

Chronic skin conditions may develop as a result of ongoing mast cell activation. These can include eczema-like rashes, chronic urticaria, or other inflammatory skin conditions that don't respond well to conventional dermatological treatments.

Lisa, a 29-year-old teacher, experienced skin-dominant MCAS: "My skin became my enemy. I would break out in hives from things that never bothered me before - my laundry detergent, perfumes, even stress. I had to completely overhaul my skincare routine and became very careful about what products I used. The worst part was the unpredictability - I never knew when my skin would decide to react to something."

The triggers for skin-dominant MCAS include topical exposures like cosmetics, fragrances, fabrics, and cleaning products, but can also include systemic triggers like foods, medications, stress, and environmental factors. The skin often serves as a visible indicator of systemic mast cell activation, with skin symptoms accompanying internal reactions.

Diagnosis of skin-dominant MCAS may involve patch testing, photodermatitis testing, or other dermatological evaluations to rule out allergic contact dermatitis or other skin conditions. Skin biopsies may show increased numbers of mast cells or evidence of mast cell activation, though this isn't always present.

Treatment approaches include identifying and avoiding topical triggers, using gentle, fragrance-free skincare products, and applying topical treatments that can stabilize mast cells or reduce inflammation. Systemic treatments for MCAS often improve skin symptoms as well, demonstrating the connection between skin reactions and systemic mast cell activation.

Multi-System MCAS

Many patients experience symptoms involving multiple organ systems simultaneously, creating complex clinical presentations that can be challenging to diagnose and manage. Multi-system MCAS represents the most common presentation of the condition, though patients may have one predominant system that's more severely affected.

The hallmark of multi-system MCAS is the occurrence of symptoms in at least two different organ systems, often triggered by the same exposures or occurring during the same time periods. For example, a patient might experience gastrointestinal cramping, skin flushing, heart palpitations, and brain fog all during the same reaction episode.

Symptom clustering helps distinguish MCAS from multiple separate conditions. When symptoms from different body systems occur together consistently, it suggests a common underlying mechanism rather than coincidental separate diseases. Patients often notice that their "good days" and "bad days" affect multiple symptoms simultaneously.

Trigger consistency across systems provides additional evidence for MCAS. The same trigger that causes digestive symptoms might also trigger skin reactions and neurological symptoms. This consistency helps patients identify their personal trigger patterns and supports the diagnosis of a systemic condition.

Treatment response patterns in multi-system MCAS often show improvement across multiple symptoms when effective mast cell treatments are implemented. This coordinated response provides additional evidence that the symptoms share a common mechanism.

David, a 42-year-old accountant, describes his multi-system experience: "When I have a reaction, it's like my whole body goes haywire. I'll get stomach cramps, my heart starts racing, my skin gets red and itchy, and I can't think clearly. It usually starts with one symptom, and then others follow within minutes. My doctors initially thought I had multiple separate conditions until someone realized they were all connected."

The complexity of multi-system MCAS requires coordinated care that addresses the underlying mast cell activation while managing specific symptoms in different organ systems. This often involves working with multiple specialists who understand the connections between the various symptoms.

Common Comorbidities and Overlapping Conditions

MCAS frequently occurs alongside other conditions, either as a result of chronic inflammation and mast cell activation or due to shared underlying mechanisms. Understanding these associations helps patients and healthcare providers recognize the full scope of health issues that may need to be addressed.

Autoimmune conditions appear to occur more frequently in people with MCAS than in the general population. The chronic inflammation caused by mast cell activation may trigger autoimmune responses, or there may be shared genetic factors that predispose individuals to both types of conditions. Common autoimmune comorbidities include thyroid disorders, rheumatoid arthritis, and inflammatory bowel diseases.

Allergic conditions often coexist with MCAS, though they represent different mechanisms of immune system activation. Food allergies, environmental allergies, and asthma may be more severe or difficult to manage in patients with underlying MCAS. The presence of multiple allergic conditions sometimes leads to the discovery of underlying mast cell activation.

Postural orthostatic tachycardia syndrome (POTS) and other forms of dysautonomia frequently occur with MCAS. The inflammation caused by mast cell activation can affect the autonomic nervous system, leading to problems with heart rate, blood pressure regulation, and other autonomic functions.

Ehlers-Danlos syndrome and other connective tissue disorders show a significant association with MCAS. The exact relationship isn't fully understood, but both conditions may share genetic factors or the connective tissue abnormalities in EDS may predispose to mast cell activation.

Mental health conditions including anxiety and depression may be more common in MCAS patients. While some of these symptoms may be direct effects of mast cell mediators on the brain, others may be secondary to the stress and impact of living with a chronic, unpredictable condition.

Dr. Andrew, a rheumatologist who treats many patients with complex multi-system conditions, notes: "When I see a patient with multiple conditions that seem unrelated - maybe they have POTS, some autoimmune markers, recurrent infections, and digestive issues - I always consider the possibility of underlying MCAS. Treating the mast cell activation often improves multiple seemingly separate conditions."

Understanding these associations helps patients advocate for appropriate evaluation and treatment of comorbid conditions. It also helps explain why comprehensive care often requires addressing multiple health issues simultaneously rather than focusing on individual symptoms or diagnoses.

The recognition of comorbidities also influences treatment decisions, as some medications used for MCAS may also benefit associated conditions, while others might worsen comorbid issues. This complexity requires careful coordination between healthcare providers and individualized treatment approaches.

Embracing Your Unique Pattern

Understanding your personal MCAS phenotype transforms your relationship with your symptoms from confusion and fear to knowledge and empowerment. Your unique pattern of symptoms, triggers, and responses isn't a puzzle to be solved once and forgotten - it's a dynamic map that guides your daily decisions and long-term health strategies.

This personalized understanding becomes the foundation for everything that follows in your MCAS management journey. Instead of trying to fit your experience into someone else's story, you can develop strategies that work specifically for your body, your triggers, and your life circumstances. Your pattern may evolve over time, but the skills you develop in recognizing and responding to your unique presentation will serve you throughout that evolution.

The diversity of MCAS presentations demonstrates that there's no single "right" way to experience this condition. Your symptoms are valid regardless of how they compare to others, and your management needs are unique to your situation. This understanding frees you to focus on what works for you rather than comparing your experience to others or feeling like you should respond to treatments the same way as other patients.

Key Learning Points

- MCAS presents differently in each person, with symptoms ranging from mild to severe across various body systems

- Gastrointestinal, cardiovascular, neurological, and skin-dominant presentations each have characteristic features and triggers

- Multi-system involvement is common and helps distinguish MCAS from other single-system conditions

- Comorbid conditions frequently occur with MCAS and may share underlying mechanisms or result from chronic inflammation

- Recognizing your personal phenotype guides treatment decisions and helps predict responses to interventions

- Understanding symptom patterns and trigger relationships forms the foundation for effective long-term management

Chapter 4: Environmental Trigger Management

- Creating Your Safe Spaces

The scent hits you before you even realize what's happening. Walking through the department store, you suddenly feel that familiar tightness in your chest, the flush creeping up your neck, and the unmistakable warning signs that your mast cells are gearing up for action. You hadn't planned to react to anything today - you just needed to pick up a birthday gift - but your body has other ideas. This scenario plays out countless times for people with MCAS, turning everyday environments into potential minefields of unexpected triggers.

Your environment plays a powerful role in your MCAS management, far beyond what most people realize. The air you breathe, the products you use, the spaces you occupy, and even the weather conditions can all influence your mast cell stability. Learning to identify, modify, and control these environmental factors becomes one of your most powerful tools for maintaining wellness and preventing reactions.

Common Environmental Triggers

Understanding the broad categories of environmental triggers helps you develop awareness and protective strategies. These triggers don't affect everyone with MCAS equally, but knowing what to watch for allows you to identify your personal sensitivities and take appropriate precautions.

Chemical exposures represent one of the most significant categories of environmental triggers. Volatile organic compounds (VOCs) from cleaning products, paints, adhesives, and building materials can activate mast cells even at concentrations that don't bother most people. These chemicals become airborne and can trigger reactions through inhalation, skin contact, or even absorption through clothing (10).

Fragrances deserve special attention because they're ubiquitous in modern environments. Perfumes, air fresheners, scented candles, laundry products, and personal care items all contain complex mixtures of synthetic chemicals designed to smell appealing. For people with MCAS, these same chemicals can trigger immediate reactions or contribute to overall mast cell instability.

Temperature extremes can directly activate mast cells through physical mechanisms. Heat exposure causes vasodilation and can trigger flushing, heart palpitations, and other cardiovascular symptoms. Cold exposure can cause different types of mast cell activation, sometimes leading to hives, joint pain, or respiratory symptoms. The key is recognizing your individual temperature tolerance and planning accordingly.

Humidity levels affect both comfort and mast cell stability. High humidity can worsen symptoms in some people while helping others. Low humidity can dry out mucous membranes and make them more reactive to other triggers. Many patients find they have an optimal humidity range where they feel most stable.

Air quality factors including pollution, allergens, and particulate matter can trigger MCAS reactions. Poor air quality from traffic, industrial sources, or natural causes like wildfire smoke can activate mast cells in sensitive individuals. Even indoor air quality issues like dust, mold, or poor ventilation can contribute to symptom flares.

Patricia, a 45-year-old librarian, learned to recognize her environmental patterns: "I started tracking my symptoms along with weather conditions and realized that high pollution days were always bad for me. I also noticed that certain areas of the library triggered my symptoms - turns out there was a mold problem in the basement archives that was affecting the air quality throughout the building."

Electromagnetic fields remain a controversial trigger, but some MCAS patients report sensitivity to WiFi, cell phone signals, or other electronic devices. The research on this connection is limited, but individual experiences suggest that some people benefit from reducing exposure to electromagnetic radiation.

Barometric pressure changes associated with weather fronts can trigger symptoms in sensitive individuals. Many patients report feeling worse before storms or during rapid weather changes. This connection likely relates to the physical effects of pressure changes on mast cells and blood vessels.

Home Environment Optimization

Your home should be your sanctuary - a place where you can control exposures and minimize triggers. Creating an MCAS-friendly home environment requires systematic attention to air quality, chemical exposures, and physical comfort factors.

Air quality improvement starts with identifying and eliminating sources of indoor air pollution. Replace standard cleaning products with fragrance-free, chemical-free alternatives. Remove air fresheners, scented candles, and other sources of synthetic fragrances. Consider switching to unscented personal care products and laundry detergents.

High-quality air filtration can make a dramatic difference in symptom control. HEPA air purifiers remove particles, allergens, and some chemical vapors from indoor air. Place units in bedrooms and main living areas for maximum benefit. Some patients find that whole-house filtration systems or upgraded HVAC filters provide additional protection.

Chemical reduction strategies extend beyond cleaning products to include building materials, furniture, and fabrics. New carpets, furniture, and paint can off-gas chemicals for months or years. Choose low-VOC or no-VOC paints, adhesives, and building materials when possible. Natural fiber furnishings generally emit fewer chemicals than synthetic materials.

The bedroom deserves special attention since you spend eight hours or more each day in this space. Use organic cotton or bamboo bedding, avoid flame retardants in mattresses and pillows, and ensure good ventilation. Some patients benefit from air purifiers specifically designed for bedrooms.

Temperature and humidity control helps maintain optimal conditions for mast cell stability. Consistent temperatures reduce thermal stress, while humidity control prevents mold growth and maintains comfortable conditions. Many patients find that slightly cool, moderately humid conditions work best for them.

Mark, a 38-year-old accountant, transformed his home environment: "I went through every room systematically, replacing cleaning products, removing air fresheners, and adding air purifiers. The biggest difference was switching to fragrance-free everything - laundry detergent, soap, shampoo, even toilet paper. It took about six months to complete the transformation, but my daily symptoms improved dramatically."

Storage and organization strategies help minimize dust accumulation and make cleaning easier. Reduce clutter that can collect dust and particles. Use sealed storage containers for items that might outgas chemicals. Keep frequently used items in easy-to-clean areas to reduce exposure to cleaning products.

Pet considerations require special attention for MCAS patients. Pet dander, saliva, and urine can trigger reactions in sensitive individuals. Regular grooming, air filtration, and keeping pets out of bedrooms can help reduce exposures while allowing you to enjoy animal companionship.

Workplace Modifications

Spending eight or more hours daily in a workplace environment makes it critical to address potential triggers in this setting. Unlike your home, you may have limited control over workplace conditions, but understanding your rights and communicating effectively with employers can help create a safer work environment.

Indoor air quality in office buildings often poses challenges for MCAS patients. Poor ventilation, chemical cleaning products, air fresheners, and off-gassing from office furniture and equipment can create trigger-rich environments. Building maintenance activities like carpet cleaning, painting, or pest control can temporarily worsen air quality.

Fragrance policies can provide significant protection for chemically sensitive employees. Many workplaces now recognize fragrance sensitivity as a legitimate health concern and implement fragrance-free policies. These policies typically request that employees avoid wearing perfumes, colognes, and heavily scented personal care products.

Personal workspace modifications allow you to create a safer microenvironment within your work area. Small desktop air purifiers can improve local air quality. Natural fiber clothing can reduce static and chemical exposure. Bringing your own cleaning supplies for your workspace allows you to avoid triggering chemicals.

Communication strategies with supervisors and human resources help ensure your needs are understood and accommodated. Focus on specific, reasonable requests rather than general complaints about air quality. Document your symptoms and their relationship to workplace exposures to support accommodation requests.

Lisa, a 32-year-old marketing manager, successfully advocated for workplace changes: "I approached HR with specific suggestions rather than just complaining about feeling sick at work. I requested that they stop using air fresheners in our department, switch to fragrance-free cleaning products in my area, and allow me to use a small air purifier at my desk. They were surprisingly receptive once I explained that these were medical accommodations."

Remote work considerations have become more common and can provide significant benefits for MCAS patients. Working from home allows complete control over your environment and eliminates commute-related exposures. Many employers now offer flexible work arrangements that can reduce symptom severity.

Travel between locations within your workplace can expose you to different air quality conditions. Elevators, stairwells, parking garages, and other building areas may have different ventilation or chemical exposures. Planning routes and timing can help minimize problematic exposures.

Air Quality Management

Air quality management forms the foundation of environmental trigger control for most MCAS patients. Understanding air quality factors and implementing appropriate controls can significantly reduce daily symptom burden and prevent acute reactions.

Outdoor air quality monitoring helps you plan activities and adjust precautions based on current conditions. Air quality indices report levels of particulate matter, ozone, and other pollutants that can trigger MCAS symptoms. Many weather apps now include air quality information, and specialized apps provide detailed pollution data.

High pollution days require modified activities and increased precautions. Stay indoors when possible, keep windows closed, and use air conditioning with recirculation settings. If you must go outside, consider wearing a high-quality mask designed to filter particles and some chemical vapors.

Indoor air quality testing can identify specific problems in your home or workplace. Professional testing can detect mold, VOCs, formaldehyde, and other potential triggers. Home testing kits provide basic information about common indoor air pollutants, though professional testing offers more detailed analysis.

Ventilation strategies help remove pollutants and bring in fresh air when outdoor conditions permit. Natural ventilation through windows and doors works well when outdoor air quality is good. Mechanical ventilation systems should include appropriate filtration to remove outdoor pollutants.

Air filtration technology has advanced significantly in recent years, offering better options for people with chemical sensitivities. HEPA filters remove particles but don't address chemical vapors. Activated carbon filters absorb many chemicals but need regular replacement. Combined HEPA and carbon filtration systems address both particles and chemicals.

Some patients benefit from more advanced filtration technologies like photocatalytic oxidation or ionization, though these technologies can produce ozone or other byproducts that may trigger sensitive individuals. Test any new filtration system carefully to ensure it helps rather than worsens your symptoms.

Dr. Jennifer, an environmental medicine physician, explains: "I recommend that MCAS patients start with basic air quality improvements - eliminate obvious sources, add HEPA filtration, and monitor outdoor air quality. Advanced technologies can help some people, but the basics often provide the most significant improvement."

Chemical Avoidance Strategies

Modern life exposes us to thousands of synthetic chemicals daily, many of which can trigger mast cell activation in sensitive individuals. Developing effective chemical avoidance strategies requires understanding common sources of exposure and implementing practical alternatives.

Personal care products represent a major source of chemical exposure through direct skin contact and inhalation of vapors. Conventional shampoos, soaps, moisturizers, and cosmetics contain fragrances, preservatives, and other chemicals that can trigger reactions. Switch to fragrance-free, chemical-free alternatives or make your own products using simple, natural ingredients.

Cleaning products contribute significantly to indoor chemical exposure. Conventional cleaners contain VOCs, fragrances, and other potentially triggering compounds. Replace these with simple alternatives like white vinegar, baking soda, and castile soap. Many health food stores carry cleaning products specifically designed for chemically sensitive individuals.

Laundry products including detergents, fabric softeners, and dryer sheets can cause reactions through skin contact with treated fabrics and inhalation of residual chemicals. Fragrance-free, dye-free detergents reduce exposure. Avoid fabric softeners and dryer sheets, which leave chemical residues on clothing. White vinegar can serve as a natural fabric softener.

Food packaging and storage can introduce chemicals through direct contact with food. Plastic containers may leach chemicals, particularly when heated. Glass and stainless steel containers provide safer storage options. Avoid heating food in plastic containers or using plastic wrap in microwave ovens.

Michael, a 41-year-old teacher, simplified his chemical exposures: "I replaced all my cleaning products with just four items: white vinegar, baking soda, castile soap, and hydrogen peroxide. I can clean my entire house with these simple ingredients, and my symptoms improved dramatically once I eliminated all the conventional cleaners."

New product introductions require careful testing and gradual implementation. Introduce one new product at a time so you can identify any that trigger reactions. Test new products in small amounts or limited areas before full use. Keep detailed records of products that work well for you.

Chemical exposure reduction extends beyond product choices to include behavioral modifications. Avoid walking through perfume sections in stores. Shop during off-peak hours when fewer people are wearing fragrances. Choose seating in restaurants away from restrooms where air fresheners are common.

Travel Planning and Safety

Travel presents unique challenges for MCAS patients, exposing you to unfamiliar environments, different air quality conditions, and limited control over chemical exposures. Careful planning and preparation can help make travel safer and more enjoyable.

Accommodation selection requires research beyond typical travel considerations. Contact hotels directly to ask about their cleaning products, air fresheners, and room preparation procedures. Request rooms that haven't been recently painted or carpeted. Some hotel chains offer allergy-friendly rooms with improved air filtration and chemical-free cleaning protocols.

Transportation considerations vary depending on your mode of travel. Airlines use strong cleaning chemicals and recirculate cabin air that may contain fragrances from other passengers. Trains and buses may have poor ventilation and chemical exposures. Private vehicle travel offers the most control over your environment.

Packing strategies should include emergency supplies and familiar products. Bring your own bedding if possible, or at least pillowcases made from tolerated fabrics. Pack air purifiers designed for travel, emergency medications, and safe personal care products. Research availability of safe products at your destination in case you run out.

Destination research helps identify potential triggers and safe options at your travel location. Check air quality forecasts for your travel dates. Research local hospitals and medical facilities in case you need emergency care. Identify stores that carry safe products you might need during your trip.

Sarah, a 36-year-old nurse, developed a successful travel system: "I always pack a small air purifier, my own pillowcase, and a full set of my safe cleaning products. I call hotels in advance to request no air fresheners in my room and no fabric softener on the linens. I also research the local air quality and plan indoor activities for high pollution days."

Emergency preparedness becomes even more critical when traveling. Carry extra emergency medications and know how to access medical care at your destination. Have contact information for your healthcare providers and consider medical alert identification that mentions your MCAS diagnosis.

Emergency Environment Assessment

Sometimes you'll find yourself in environments that trigger reactions despite your best planning efforts. Learning to quickly assess and respond to problematic environments can prevent minor exposures from becoming major reactions.

Rapid trigger identification skills help you recognize problematic environments quickly. Trust your initial instincts - if you feel symptoms starting, identify and address the trigger immediately rather than hoping symptoms will resolve on their own. Common signs include increased heart rate, flushing, respiratory irritation, or cognitive changes.

Immediate response strategies can minimize reaction severity when you encounter unexpected triggers. Leave the triggering environment if possible. Remove or distance yourself from the trigger source. Take rescue medications promptly rather than waiting for symptoms to worsen.

Environmental modifications may be possible even in unfamiliar settings. Ask building management to turn off air fresheners or reduce fragrance use. Open windows for fresh air if outdoor conditions permit. Move to different areas of a building that may have different air quality.

Exit strategies should be planned before entering potentially problematic environments. Know where exits are located and have transportation arranged. Carry emergency contact information and ensure someone knows your location and expected return time.

Dr. Michael, an allergist experienced with MCAS, advises: "Patients often wait too long to leave triggering environments, hoping their symptoms will improve. The key is trusting your body's signals and taking action immediately. It's much easier to prevent a reaction than to treat one once it's started."

Building Your Environmental Foundation

Creating and maintaining safe environments requires ongoing attention and adjustment, but the investment pays tremendous dividends in improved daily comfort and reduced reaction frequency. Your environmental management skills will develop over time as you learn to recognize subtle triggers and implement effective protective strategies.

The goal isn't to live in isolation or avoid all potential exposures, but rather to reduce your overall trigger load to a manageable level while maintaining quality of life. Small, consistent improvements in your environmental conditions often provide more benefit than dramatic changes that are difficult to sustain.

Your environment serves as the foundation for all other MCAS management strategies. When your environmental trigger load is well-controlled, you'll have more resilience to handle occasional dietary indiscretions, stress, or other unavoidable triggers. This environmental stability creates space for healing and allows your other management strategies to work more effectively.

Key Learning Points

- Environmental triggers include chemical exposures, temperature extremes, air quality issues, and electromagnetic fields that can activate mast cells

- Home environment optimization focuses on air quality improvement, chemical reduction, and temperature control to create stable conditions

- Workplace modifications require communication skills and specific accommodation requests to reduce occupational exposures

- Air quality management involves monitoring outdoor conditions and implementing appropriate filtration and ventilation strategies

- Chemical avoidance requires systematic replacement of conventional products with safer alternatives and behavioral modifications

- Travel planning must account for accommodation safety, transportation exposures, and emergency preparedness in unfamiliar environments

Chapter 5: Dietary Approaches and Nutrition

- Nourishing Your Body While Managing Triggers

Standing in the grocery store with a shopping list that seems to eliminate half the foods you once enjoyed can feel overwhelming and isolating. Reading every ingredient label, questioning each meal decision, and watching others eat freely while you calculate histamine levels creates a relationship with food that goes far beyond simple nutrition. For people with MCAS, food becomes both medicine and potential trigger, requiring a careful balance between nourishment and symptom management.

The connection between food and MCAS symptoms extends beyond traditional food allergies or intolerances. Your digestive system contains large numbers of mast cells that can react to specific foods, food additives, preparation methods, and even the timing of meals. Understanding these complex relationships allows you to maintain proper nutrition while minimizing dietary triggers and optimizing your overall health.

Histamine and Dietary Triggers

Histamine plays a central role in many MCAS food reactions, but the relationship between dietary histamine and symptoms is more complex than simply avoiding high-histamine foods. Understanding histamine metabolism, individual tolerance levels, and the factors that influence histamine sensitivity helps you make informed dietary decisions.

Histamine sources in food come from both natural content and bacterial production during food processing, aging, or spoilage. Foods naturally high in histamine include aged cheeses, fermented products, cured meats, and certain fish species. Bacterial fermentation increases histamine levels in foods like sauerkraut, wine, and aged cheeses. Food spoilage also rapidly increases histamine content, making freshness particularly important for sensitive individuals (11).

Histamine liberation occurs when certain foods trigger your mast cells to release their own histamine stores, even if the food itself doesn't contain high levels of histamine. Common histamine-liberating foods include citrus fruits, tomatoes, strawberries, chocolate, nuts, and certain spices. These foods can cause reactions in sensitive individuals regardless of their actual histamine content.

Histamine degradation depends on enzymes that break down histamine in your digestive system. The primary enzyme, diamine oxidase (DAO), can be overwhelmed by high histamine loads or may be naturally low in some individuals. Alcohol, certain medications, and some foods can inhibit DAO activity, increasing your effective histamine exposure even from moderate-histamine foods (12).

Individual tolerance levels vary significantly between people and can change over time within the same individual. Factors like stress, illness, hormonal changes, and overall mast cell stability affect your histamine tolerance. Some people can tolerate moderate amounts of high-histamine foods when their mast cells are stable, while others need to maintain strict avoidance.

Jenny, a 29-year-old graphic designer, describes her histamine learning curve: "I initially tried to follow strict low-histamine lists I found online, but I was still having reactions to supposedly 'safe' foods. My nutritionist helped me understand that freshness mattered more than specific foods, and that my tolerance changed depending on my stress levels and hormonal cycle. Now I adjust my diet based on how I'm feeling overall."

Histamine accumulation can occur when you consume multiple moderate-histamine foods close together, creating a cumulative effect that triggers symptoms. This explains why you might tolerate a small amount of aged cheese one day but react to the same amount when combined with wine and tomatoes. Understanding this accumulation effect helps you space histamine-containing foods and monitor your total daily load.

Cofactor interactions influence how your body processes histamine. Vitamin B6, vitamin C, and copper are essential for proper histamine metabolism. Deficiencies in these nutrients can worsen histamine intolerance. Conversely, certain nutrients and compounds can compete with histamine metabolism, effectively increasing your histamine burden.

The Low-Histamine Diet - Basics and Implementation

The low-histamine diet serves as a foundation for many MCAS patients, though it requires careful implementation to ensure nutritional adequacy while effectively reducing symptoms. Understanding the principles behind histamine restriction helps you adapt the diet to your individual needs and circumstances.

Fresh foods form the cornerstone of a low-histamine diet. Freshly prepared meats, fish, vegetables, and fruits generally contain lower histamine levels than processed or aged alternatives. The key is minimizing the time between food preparation and consumption, as histamine levels increase with storage time, even under refrigeration.

Preparation methods significantly influence histamine content. Grilling, baking, and steaming generally produce lower histamine levels than slow-cooking methods. Avoid reheating foods multiple times, as each heating cycle can increase histamine content. Prepare smaller portions that you'll consume immediately rather than making large batches for leftovers.

Storage strategies help maintain low histamine levels in fresh foods. Freeze foods you won't use immediately to prevent histamine accumulation. Use fresh or frozen vegetables rather than canned versions when possible. Store opened packages properly and use them quickly to prevent bacterial growth that increases histamine production.

Protein sources require particular attention since many high-protein foods are also high in histamine. Fresh fish and poultry generally work well for most people, but avoid aged, cured, or processed meats. Some people tolerate certain fish better than others - salmon and sardines are often well-tolerated, while tuna and mackerel may cause problems due to higher natural histamine content.

Vegetable and fruit selections focus on those with lower natural histamine content and minimal histamine-liberating properties. Well-tolerated vegetables often include broccoli, cauliflower, zucchini, carrots, and leafy greens. Fruits like apples, pears, and melons are often safer choices than citrus fruits, berries, or tropical fruits.

David, a 44-year-old engineer, found success with systematic implementation: "I started with a very basic low-histamine diet for two weeks - just fresh chicken, rice, broccoli, and apples. Once my symptoms stabilized, I slowly added one new food every few days to see what I could tolerate. It took about three months to build up a reasonable variety of foods I could eat safely."

Meal timing can influence histamine tolerance in some individuals. Eating smaller, more frequent meals may be better tolerated than large meals. Some people find that histamine tolerance varies throughout the day, with better tolerance in the morning than evening. Pay attention to your individual patterns and adjust meal timing accordingly.

Cooking techniques can help reduce histamine content and improve tolerance. Blanching vegetables before cooking can reduce some natural compounds that might trigger reactions. Using fresh herbs instead of dried spices often works better for sensitive individuals. Simple preparation methods with minimal ingredients help identify problem foods more easily.

Elimination Diet Protocols

Elimination diets provide a systematic approach to identifying specific food triggers beyond general histamine considerations. These protocols require patience and careful documentation but can provide invaluable information about your individual dietary tolerances and optimal nutrition plan.

Planning phase involves selecting an appropriate elimination protocol based on your symptoms, suspected triggers, and nutritional needs. Basic elimination diets remove common trigger foods for 2-4 weeks while maintaining adequate nutrition. More extensive protocols may eliminate multiple food categories simultaneously, though these require careful nutritional planning.

Common elimination targets include histamine-rich foods, common allergens (eggs, dairy, wheat, soy, nuts), food additives, artificial colors and flavors, preservatives, and foods known to trigger mast cell activation. Some protocols also eliminate nightshade vegetables, FODMAPs, or other specific food categories based on individual symptoms.

Baseline establishment requires 2-4 weeks of strict adherence to your elimination diet. This period allows your immune system to calm down and provides a stable baseline for evaluating food reintroductions. Document your symptoms carefully during this phase to establish your improved symptom levels.

Support strategies help ensure success during the restrictive elimination phase. Meal planning and preparation become critical when your food options are limited. Consider working with a nutritionist familiar with elimination diets to ensure nutritional adequacy. Having family support and understanding makes the process much more manageable.

Lisa, a 33-year-old teacher, shares her elimination experience: "The hardest part was the social isolation - I couldn't eat out with friends or enjoy family meals for several weeks. But tracking my symptoms carefully showed me just how much certain foods were affecting my daily functioning.

The information I gained was worth the temporary restrictions."

Documentation methods should capture both food intake and symptom patterns. Food diaries should include exact foods eaten, portion sizes, preparation methods, and timing. Symptom logs should track intensity, timing, and duration of reactions. Some people find that apps or spreadsheets help organize this information effectively.

Success indicators include reduced symptom frequency and intensity, improved energy levels, better sleep quality, and stabilization of previously fluctuating symptoms. Not everyone will achieve complete symptom resolution during elimination phases, but most people notice some improvement if food triggers are contributing to their symptoms.

Food Reintroduction Strategies

The reintroduction phase of elimination diets provides specific information about individual food tolerances and helps expand your diet while maintaining symptom control. Systematic reintroduction requires patience and careful monitoring but allows you to identify specific problematic foods rather than unnecessarily restricting your entire diet.

Reintroduction timing should begin only after you've achieved a stable symptom baseline during the elimination phase. Most practitioners recommend waiting at least 2-4 weeks of stable symptoms before beginning reintroductions. Starting too early can make it difficult to distinguish between elimination diet benefits and reintroduction reactions.

Systematic approach involves introducing one food at a time in sufficient quantities to trigger a reaction if you're sensitive to that food. Eat the test food 2-3 times during one day, then wait 2-3 days before introducing the next food. This spacing allows time for delayed reactions to develop and clear before testing the next food.

Quantity considerations require eating enough of the test food to trigger a reaction if you're sensitive to it. Small tastes may not provide sufficient exposure to identify problems. However, start with moderate portions rather than large amounts to avoid severe reactions if you are sensitive to the food.

Reaction assessment involves monitoring for both immediate and delayed symptoms. Immediate reactions occur within minutes to hours and are usually easy to identify. Delayed reactions can occur up to 72 hours after eating a food and may be more subtle. Track symptoms like energy changes, mood changes, sleep disturbances, and digestive symptoms in addition to obvious allergic reactions.

Mark, a 39-year-old accountant, developed an effective reintroduction system: "I kept a detailed symptom diary and photographed every meal during reintroduction. When I reacted to a food, I could look back at exactly what I ate and how much. I discovered that I could tolerate small amounts of some foods that caused problems in larger quantities."

Priority ordering helps you test the most important foods first. Start with foods you miss most or that would significantly improve your diet quality if tolerated. Consider nutritional value when prioritizing - reintroducing tolerated protein sources or nutrient-dense vegetables may be more valuable than testing dessert foods.

Retesting considerations may be appropriate for foods that initially caused reactions. Food tolerances can change over time as your overall health improves. Some people find they can reintroduce previously problematic foods after several months of good mast cell stability.

Nutritional Deficiencies and Supplementation

Restrictive diets necessary for MCAS management can lead to nutritional deficiencies if not carefully planned. Understanding common deficiency risks and implementing appropriate supplementation helps maintain optimal health while managing food triggers.

Common deficiency risks in MCAS patients include B vitamins (particularly B12, folate, and B6), vitamin D, iron, magnesium, zinc, and essential fatty acids. These deficiencies can result from restrictive diets, poor absorption due to intestinal inflammation, or increased needs due to chronic inflammation and stress (13).

B vitamin deficiencies are particularly common because many B vitamin-rich foods are restricted on low-histamine diets. B12 deficiency can worsen neurological symptoms and fatigue. Folate deficiency affects energy metabolism and mood. B6 deficiency can worsen histamine intolerance since B6 is required for histamine metabolism.

Mineral deficiencies can develop gradually and may worsen MCAS symptoms. Magnesium deficiency can increase anxiety, muscle tension, and sleep problems. Zinc deficiency affects immune function and wound healing. Iron deficiency causes fatigue and can worsen exercise intolerance.

Fat-soluble vitamin status requires attention since many MCAS patients avoid dairy products and may have fat malabsorption issues. Vitamin D deficiency is common and can worsen immune dysfunction. Vitamin K deficiency can affect blood clotting, which may be particularly relevant for patients taking anticoagulant medications.

Dr. Sarah, a nutritionist specializing in elimination diets, explains: "I see many MCAS patients who develop nutritional deficiencies because they're afraid to eat diverse foods. The key is working systematically to identify truly problematic foods while maintaining as varied a diet as possible. Strategic supplementation can bridge nutritional gaps during restrictive phases."

Testing protocols help identify specific deficiencies before they cause symptoms. Basic nutritional panels should include B12, folate, iron studies, vitamin D, and magnesium. More extensive testing might include amino acid profiles, fatty acid analysis, and organic acid testing to assess metabolic function.

Supplementation strategies must account for potential sensitivities to supplement ingredients. Many supplements contain fillers, colors, or preservatives that can trigger MCAS reactions. Choose high-quality supplements with minimal ingredients, or consider compounding pharmacies that can prepare custom formulations without problematic additives.

Meal Planning and Preparation

Successful MCAS dietary management requires systematic meal planning and preparation to ensure adequate nutrition while avoiding triggers. Developing efficient systems reduces daily decision-making stress and helps maintain dietary consistency.

Weekly planning helps ensure nutritional balance and reduces daily food-related stress. Plan meals around well-tolerated foods, incorporating variety within your safe food list. Consider your schedule when planning - prepare simpler meals for busy days and more elaborate meals when you have more time and energy.

Batch preparation can save time while maintaining food freshness. Prepare larger quantities of well-tolerated base ingredients like grains, proteins, and vegetables that you can combine in different ways throughout the week. Freeze individual portions to maintain freshness and prevent histamine accumulation.

Fresh ingredient focus becomes particularly important when managing histamine sensitivity. Shop more frequently for fresh produce rather than relying on long-term storage. Build relationships with local farmers or markets that can provide information about harvest dates and storage methods.

Kitchen organization supports efficient meal preparation and reduces contamination risks. Store safe foods separately from potentially problematic ones. Use glass containers for storage to avoid chemical leaching from plastics. Label prepared foods with dates to track freshness.

Jennifer, a 31-year-old nurse, developed an efficient system: "I spend Sunday mornings preparing base ingredients for the week - cooking grains, washing and chopping vegetables, and preparing proteins. During the week, I just combine these ingredients in different ways. It saves time and ensures I always have safe foods available when I'm tired after work."

Recipe adaptation allows you to enjoy familiar foods using safe ingredients. Learn substitution strategies for common trigger ingredients. Develop a collection of reliable recipes using your tolerated foods. Share successful adaptations with other MCAS patients to expand everyone's meal options.

Emergency meal planning ensures you have safe options available during symptom flares or busy periods. Keep ingredients for simple, quick meals that you know you tolerate well. Consider shelf-stable options that don't require fresh preparation when you're feeling unwell.

Dining Out and Social Eating

Maintaining social connections around food requires careful planning and communication skills, but it's possible to participate in social eating while managing MCAS dietary needs. Developing strategies for restaurant dining and social events helps maintain quality of life and relationships.

Restaurant research should begin before you arrive at the restaurant. Call ahead to discuss your dietary needs and ask about ingredient lists, preparation methods, and cross-contamination prevention. Many restaurants can accommodate special dietary needs if given advance notice.

Menu navigation requires understanding how foods are prepared and what ingredients might be hidden in dishes. Ask detailed questions about seasonings, marinades, sauces, and cooking methods. Simple preparations are often safer than complex dishes with multiple ingredients.

Communication strategies with restaurant staff should be clear but not overly complex. Focus on specific foods you need to avoid rather than trying to explain MCAS. Emphasize that your restrictions are medical requirements, not preferences. Consider bringing a restaurant card that lists your main dietary restrictions.

Safe backup plans help ensure you have eating options even if the restaurant can't accommodate your needs. Research backup restaurants in the area. Consider eating a small meal before going out so you're not hungry if safe options aren't available. Bring safe snacks if appropriate for the social situation.

Michael, a 35-year-old marketing manager, shares his dining strategies: "I learned to call restaurants during slow periods when staff have time to discuss ingredients. I always have a backup plan - either another restaurant nearby or snacks in my car. I've found that most places are very accommodating when they understand it's a medical issue."

Social event navigation requires balancing your dietary needs with social participation. Offer to bring a dish you can eat to potluck events. Eat beforehand if you're unsure about food options. Focus on the social aspects of gatherings rather than making food the center of attention.

Travel considerations extend dining challenges to unfamiliar locations. Research restaurants at your destination before traveling. Consider accommodations with kitchen facilities so you can prepare some of your own meals. Pack emergency safe foods for situations where suitable options aren't available.

Nourishing Your Body and Soul

Managing MCAS through dietary approaches requires more than just avoiding trigger foods - it's about developing a sustainable relationship with food that nourishes both your body and your spirit. The restrictions may seem overwhelming at first, but most people find that their improved health and energy levels make the dietary changes worthwhile.

Your dietary journey with MCAS will be unique to your individual triggers, tolerances, and preferences. The goal is finding the optimal balance between symptom management and quality of life, allowing you to maintain proper nutrition while participating in social activities and enjoying your meals. This balance may shift over time as your condition stabilizes and your tolerances change.

The knowledge you gain about your individual food triggers and nutritional needs becomes a powerful tool for long-term health management. Understanding how foods affect your symptoms allows you to make informed decisions about when strict adherence is necessary and when you might choose to accept mild symptoms for social or emotional benefits.

Key Learning Points

- Histamine in food comes from natural content, bacterial fermentation, and food spoilage, with individual tolerance levels varying significantly

- Low-histamine diets focus on fresh foods, proper storage, and simple preparation methods to minimize histamine exposure

- Elimination diets provide systematic approaches to identifying specific food triggers beyond general histamine considerations

- Food reintroduction requires careful timing, systematic approach, and detailed symptom monitoring to identify individual tolerances

- Nutritional deficiencies are common risks that require monitoring and strategic supplementation during restrictive dietary phases

- Meal planning and preparation systems help maintain nutritional adequacy while managing time and energy constraints

- Social eating situations require advance planning, clear communication, and backup strategies to maintain relationships while managing dietary restrictions

Chapter 6: Medication Protocols and Management

- Your Pharmaceutical Toolkit

The pharmacy counter can feel like a battlefield when you're picking up yet another prescription, hoping this one will finally provide the relief you've been seeking. Your medicine cabinet may already overflow with antihistamines, supplements, and rescue medications, each representing hope for better symptom control. For people with MCAS, medications serve multiple roles - preventing reactions, managing acute symptoms, and supporting overall mast cell stability - but finding the right combination requires patience, careful monitoring, and often some trial and error.

Medication management in MCAS goes beyond simply taking pills when symptoms occur. Your pharmaceutical toolkit needs to address the complex, multi-system nature of mast cell activation while minimizing side effects and drug interactions. Understanding how different medications work, when to use them, and how to optimize their effectiveness becomes essential for successful long-term management.

First-Line MCAS Medications

The foundation of MCAS pharmaceutical management rests on medications that directly target mast cell activation or block the effects of mast cell mediators. These first-line treatments form the backbone of most successful treatment protocols, though individual responses vary significantly.

Antihistamines represent the most commonly prescribed first-line treatments for MCAS. These medications work by blocking histamine receptors, preventing histamine from causing symptoms even when mast cells release it. The key is understanding that effective MCAS management often requires blocking multiple types of histamine receptors simultaneously.

Mast cell stabilizers work by preventing mast cells from releasing their mediators in the first place. Unlike antihistamines, which block the effects of mediators after they're released, mast cell stabilizers address the problem at its source. These medications can provide significant benefit for many patients but often take several weeks to reach full effectiveness.

Combination therapy using multiple first-line medications simultaneously often provides better symptom control than single medications alone. Most patients require at least two different types of medications to achieve optimal stability. The goal is finding the minimum effective combination that provides good symptom control with tolerable side effects.

Dr. Patricia, an immunologist specializing in MCAS, explains her approach: "I typically start patients on a combination of H1 and H2 antihistamines along with a mast cell stabilizer. This triple approach addresses histamine effects at different receptors while also reducing overall mediator release. Most patients see significant improvement within 4-6 weeks of starting this foundation regimen."

Dosing considerations for MCAS often differ from standard dosing recommendations for other conditions. Many patients require higher than typical doses or more frequent dosing to achieve symptom control. Some medications work better when taken around the clock rather than just when symptoms occur. Working with knowledgeable healthcare providers helps optimize dosing for your individual needs.

Timing strategies can significantly influence medication effectiveness. Taking antihistamines before known trigger exposures can prevent reactions more effectively than waiting until symptoms develop. Some patients benefit from splitting daily doses to maintain more consistent blood levels throughout the day.

Sarah, a 42-year-old teacher, describes finding her optimal regimen: "It took about six months of adjustments to find the right combination. I started with basic antihistamines but still had breakthrough symptoms. Adding a mast cell stabilizer made a huge difference, and we eventually found that taking my H1 antihistamine twice daily instead of once gave me much better coverage."

H1 and H2 Antihistamines

Understanding the different types of histamine receptors and the medications that block them helps you work more effectively with your healthcare provider to optimize your antihistamine regimen. Most successful MCAS protocols include both H1 and H2 antihistamines, since histamine can cause different symptoms through different receptor types.

H1 antihistamines block the histamine receptors responsible for many classic allergic symptoms. These include itching, hives, nasal congestion, sneezing, and some gastrointestinal symptoms. H1 antihistamines are further divided into first-generation and second-generation medications, each with distinct advantages and disadvantages.

First-generation H1 antihistamines like diphenhydramine (Benadryl), hydroxyzine, and chlorpheniramine cross the blood-brain barrier and can cause significant sedation. However, this sedating effect can be beneficial for patients who have trouble sleeping due to MCAS symptoms. These medications also tend to have stronger anti-inflammatory effects than newer alternatives.

Second-generation H1 antihistamines including loratadine (Claritin), cetirizine (Zyrtec), fexofenadine (Allegra), and desloratadine (Clarinex) cause less sedation because they don't readily cross the blood-brain barrier. Many patients find these more suitable for daytime use, though some people need higher than standard doses for optimal MCAS control.

H2 antihistamines block histamine receptors primarily found in the stomach and cardiovascular system. Famotidine (Pepcid) and ranitidine (though ranitidine was removed from the market due to contamination concerns) are the most commonly used H2 blockers for MCAS. These medications help with gastrointestinal symptoms and may also reduce cardiovascular symptoms like flushing and rapid heart rate (14).

Combination protocols using both H1 and H2 antihistamines often provide superior symptom control compared to either type alone. A typical regimen might include a second-generation H1 antihistamine twice daily along with an H2 antihistamine twice daily. Some patients add a first-generation H1 antihistamine at bedtime for additional coverage and sleep support.

Individual response variations mean that finding the optimal antihistamine combination requires some experimentation. Some people respond better to specific H1 antihistamines - cetirizine might work well for one person while fexofenadine works better for another. Generic versus brand name medications can also make a difference for some sensitive individuals.

Mark, a 38-year-old engineer, found his optimal combination: "I tried several different H1 antihistamines before finding that cetirizine worked best for me. Adding famotidine made a huge difference in my stomach symptoms. I take cetirizine in the morning and evening, famotidine twice daily, and add some Benadryl at night if I've had a rough day."

Dosing flexibility allows for adjustment based on symptom severity and trigger exposure. Some patients use higher doses during high-risk periods like travel or seasonal changes. Others find that they can reduce doses during stable periods. Work with your healthcare provider to develop a flexible dosing strategy that matches your individual patterns.

Mast Cell Stabilizers

Mast cell stabilizers offer a different approach to MCAS management by preventing mast cell degranulation rather than blocking the effects of released mediators. These medications can provide significant long-term benefit but require patience since they often take several weeks to reach full effectiveness.

Cromolyn sodium is the most commonly used mast cell stabilizer for MCAS. Available as an oral solution, nasal spray, and inhaler, cromolyn works by stabilizing mast cell membranes and preventing mediator release. The oral form is most commonly used for systemic MCAS, though some patients benefit from using multiple forms simultaneously.

Dosing and administration of oral cromolyn requires attention to timing and food interactions. The medication works best when taken on an empty stomach, typically 30 minutes before meals. Standard dosing is usually four times daily, though some patients need higher doses or more frequent administration. The liquid formulation can be mixed with water or juice if the taste is problematic.

Ketotifen is another mast cell stabilizer that's available in some countries but requires compounding in others. Some patients who don't respond well to cromolyn find ketotifen more effective. Ketotifen also has antihistamine properties, providing dual benefits for some patients.

Quercetin is a natural flavonoid with mast cell stabilizing properties. While not as potent as prescription mast cell stabilizers, quercetin can provide additional support and may be particularly useful for patients who can't tolerate prescription medications. Some patients use quercetin as adjunctive therapy along with prescription stabilizers.

Dr. Jennifer, an allergist experienced with mast cell stabilizers, notes: "Cromolyn is often underutilized because it takes time to work and requires frequent dosing. Patients who stick with it for at least 6-8 weeks often see significant improvement in their baseline stability. It's particularly helpful for gastrointestinal symptoms and overall trigger tolerance."

Response timeline for mast cell stabilizers typically shows gradual improvement over several weeks. Some patients notice initial benefits within days, while others require 4-6 weeks to see significant improvement. The key is maintaining consistent dosing during this buildup period, even if initial benefits aren't immediately apparent.

Combination benefits often emerge when mast cell stabilizers are used along with antihistamines. The stabilizers reduce overall mediator release while antihistamines block the effects of any mediators that are still released. This dual approach can provide more consistent symptom control than either type of medication alone.

Lisa, a 35-year-old nurse, describes her cromolyn experience: "I almost gave up on cromolyn after two weeks because I didn't notice much difference. My doctor encouraged me to continue for at least six weeks. Around week four, I suddenly realized I was having fewer reaction days overall. Now I've been on it for two years and it's made a huge difference in my baseline stability."

Rescue Medications

Rescue medications serve as your emergency response system for severe reactions or breakthrough symptoms that occur despite preventive treatments. Having an effective rescue plan and knowing how to implement it can prevent minor reactions from becoming medical emergencies.

Epinephrine auto-injectors represent the most important rescue medication for patients who experience severe reactions. While not all MCAS patients develop anaphylaxis, those who do need immediate access to epinephrine. Even patients who haven't had anaphylactic reactions may benefit from carrying epinephrine if they have severe multi-system reactions.

High-dose antihistamines can be used as rescue therapy for moderate reactions. Taking additional doses of your regular antihistamines or using faster-acting formulations like liquid diphenhydramine can help control escalating symptoms. Some patients carry antihistamine rescue packs with predetermined doses for different severity levels.

Corticosteroids may be prescribed for severe reactions, though they're typically reserved for emergency situations due to their side effect profile. Prednisone or methylprednisolone can help control severe inflammation and prevent biphasic reactions where symptoms return hours after initial treatment.

Bronchodilators become important rescue medications for patients who experience respiratory symptoms during reactions. Albuterol inhalers can provide rapid relief for bronchospasm and breathing difficulty. Some patients benefit from having both short-acting rescue inhalers and longer-acting preventive inhalers.

Rescue protocols should be clearly defined and easily accessible during emergencies. Work with your healthcare provider to develop written action plans that specify which medications to use for different symptom severities. Include dosing instructions, timing between medications, and criteria for seeking emergency medical care.

Michael, a 41-year-old accountant, developed a comprehensive rescue plan: "I carry a rescue kit everywhere with epinephrine, extra antihistamines, and my albuterol inhaler. I have written instructions for different severity levels - when to take extra antihistamines, when to use the epi-pen, and when to call 911. Having this plan written down helps me think clearly during reactions."

Emergency medical communication requires preparing information that emergency responders can understand quickly. Medical alert bracelets or cards should mention MCAS and any specific medication allergies. Consider carrying a summary of your condition, current medications, and emergency contact information.

Medication Timing and Dosing

Optimizing medication timing and dosing requires understanding how different medications work and how your symptoms fluctuate throughout the day. Strategic timing can significantly improve medication effectiveness while minimizing side effects and drug interactions.

Preventive dosing involves taking medications consistently to maintain stable blood levels rather than waiting for symptoms to develop. Most first-line MCAS medications work better when taken regularly rather than as needed. This approach helps prevent reactions rather than just treating them after they occur.

Circadian considerations account for how your symptoms and medication absorption change throughout the day. Many patients notice that symptoms are worse at certain times, often related to cortisol fluctuations, meal timing, or environmental exposures. Adjusting medication timing to anticipate these patterns can improve effectiveness.

Food interactions can affect medication absorption and effectiveness. Some medications work better on an empty stomach, while others should be taken with food to reduce gastrointestinal side effects. Cromolyn specifically requires empty stomach administration for optimal absorption.

Trigger-based timing involves adjusting medication schedules based on known trigger exposures. Taking extra antihistamines before high-risk activities, travel, or seasonal exposure periods can prevent reactions more effectively than treating them after they occur.

Dr. Sarah, a clinical pharmacist specializing in MCAS, explains: "I often see patients taking all their medications at once because it's convenient, but strategic timing can make a huge difference. Taking H1 antihistamines twice daily instead of once, or timing cromolyn before meals, can significantly improve symptom control without increasing total medication doses."

Dose escalation strategies help find the minimum effective dose for each medication. Start with standard doses and increase gradually until you achieve good symptom control. Some patients need higher than typical doses, particularly for antihistamines, to achieve optimal MCAS control.

Flexible dosing protocols allow for adjustment based on symptom severity and trigger exposure. Some patients use higher doses during unstable periods and reduce to maintenance doses during stable times. Having predetermined protocols for dose adjustments helps manage varying symptom levels effectively.

Side Effect Management

Managing medication side effects becomes particularly important for MCAS patients who often require multiple medications taken long-term. Understanding common side effects and strategies to minimize them helps maintain medication adherence while preserving quality of life.

Sedation management is especially relevant for patients taking first-generation antihistamines or higher doses of newer antihistamines. Starting with lower doses and gradually increasing can help build tolerance to sedating effects. Taking sedating medications at bedtime maximizes their sleep benefits while minimizing daytime drowsiness.

Gastrointestinal effects can occur with many MCAS medications. H2 antihistamines may cause constipation or diarrhea in some patients. Cromolyn can cause nausea or stomach upset, particularly when first starting treatment. Taking medications with small amounts of food (when appropriate) can reduce GI side effects.

Cognitive effects including brain fog or difficulty concentrating can result from some antihistamines, particularly at higher doses. If cognitive side effects are problematic, discuss alternative medications or dosing schedules with your healthcare provider. Some patients find that splitting doses reduces cognitive impact.

Cardiovascular effects may occur with certain medications, particularly in patients who already have MCAS-related cardiovascular symptoms. Monitor heart rate and blood pressure when starting new medications. Some antihistamines can cause QT prolongation, requiring ECG monitoring in high-risk patients.

Jennifer, a 39-year-old teacher, managed sedation side effects: "When I first started taking higher doses of antihistamines, I was falling asleep at my desk. My doctor suggested taking most of my dose at bedtime and a smaller dose in the morning. That solved the daytime sedation while actually improving my sleep quality."

Tolerance development can occur with some medications over time, requiring dose adjustments or medication changes. If previously effective medications seem to lose their benefit, discuss with your healthcare provider rather than simply increasing doses on your own.

Withdrawal considerations apply to some MCAS medications, particularly if they've been used long-term. Cromolyn and antihistamines generally don't cause withdrawal symptoms, but corticosteroids require gradual tapering if used for extended periods.

Drug Interactions and Contraindications

Understanding potential drug interactions becomes particularly important for MCAS patients who often take multiple medications and may have other health conditions requiring additional treatments. Some interactions can reduce medication effectiveness while others can increase side effect risks.

Antihistamine interactions can occur when multiple sedating medications are used together. Combining first-generation antihistamines with other sedating medications like sleep aids or muscle relaxants can cause excessive sedation. Alcohol can significantly increase the sedating effects of antihistamines.

Cytochrome P450 interactions affect how medications are metabolized in the liver. Some antihistamines are affected by medications that inhibit or induce these enzymes, potentially changing their effectiveness or side effect profiles. Grapefruit juice can affect some antihistamine metabolism.

QT prolongation risks can occur with certain antihistamines, particularly when combined with other medications that affect heart rhythm. Patients with cardiac conditions or those taking multiple QT-prolonging medications may need ECG monitoring.

Cromolyn interactions are generally minimal since the medication is poorly absorbed systemically. However, timing with other medications may still be important to prevent absorption issues.

Dr. Michael, a clinical pharmacist, advises: "MCAS patients often see multiple specialists who may prescribe medications without knowing about their full regimen. I recommend keeping an updated medication list and reviewing it with every healthcare provider. Some seemingly minor interactions can significantly affect symptom control."

Medical condition considerations may affect medication choices for MCAS patients. Patients with kidney disease may need dose adjustments for some antihistamines. Those with liver disease may metabolize certain medications differently. Pregnancy and breastfeeding require careful medication selection.

Supplement interactions can occur between prescription MCAS medications and natural supplements. Some supplements can increase the sedating effects of antihistamines, while others might affect medication absorption or metabolism.

Working with Pharmacists

Pharmacists represent an underutilized resource for MCAS patients navigating complex medication regimens. Developing a relationship with a knowledgeable pharmacist can significantly improve your medication management and help identify potential problems before they cause complications.

Pharmacist expertise in medication interactions, dosing, and side effects can complement your physician's care. Pharmacists often have more time to discuss medication questions and can provide detailed information about timing, food interactions, and side effect management.

Compounding services may be necessary for patients who can't tolerate commercial medication formulations due to inactive ingredients. Some patients need medications without certain dyes, preservatives, or fillers that trigger their MCAS. Compounding pharmacists can prepare customized formulations.

Insurance navigation often requires pharmacist assistance to obtain coverage for higher than typical doses or non-standard formulations. Pharmacists can help with prior authorization requests and suggest covered alternatives when preferred medications aren't covered.

Medication synchronization services help coordinate multiple prescription refills and can identify potential compliance issues. Having all medications ready at the same time reduces the risk of running out of critical medications.

Lisa, a 44-year-old marketing manager, found her pharmacist invaluable: "My pharmacist noticed that I was picking up my cromolyn prescription late every month and realized the four-times-daily dosing was hard for me to remember. She helped me set up a dosing schedule and pill organizer system that made it much easier to stay consistent."

Emergency preparedness planning with your pharmacist ensures you have access to critical medications during emergencies or travel. Discuss early refill options for rescue medications and identify 24-hour pharmacies in your area.

Medication reviews with your pharmacist can identify optimization opportunities and potential problems. Regular reviews become particularly important when medications are added or changed, or when new symptoms develop.

Building Your Medical Arsenal

Your pharmaceutical toolkit for MCAS management represents far more than a collection of medications - it's a carefully orchestrated system designed to provide stability, prevent reactions, and maintain your quality of life. Like a well-tuned instrument, this system requires regular attention and occasional adjustments to perform optimally.

The journey to finding your optimal medication regimen requires patience and persistence. What works perfectly for one person may not be suitable for another, and your own needs may change over time as your condition stabilizes or life circumstances change. The key is maintaining open communication with your healthcare team and staying committed to the process even when progress seems slow.

Your growing expertise in managing your medication regimen becomes a valuable asset in your overall MCAS care. Understanding how different medications work, recognizing side effects, and knowing when to seek adjustments empowers you to be an active participant in your treatment decisions and helps ensure the best possible outcomes from your pharmaceutical interventions.

Key Learning Points

- First-line MCAS medications include antihistamines and mast cell stabilizers that work through different mechanisms to provide symptom control

- H1 and H2 antihistamines should often be used together to block different histamine receptor types and provide better coverage

- Mast cell stabilizers prevent mediator release but require consistent dosing for several weeks to reach full effectiveness

- Rescue medications provide emergency treatment for severe reactions and should be part of a written action plan

- Medication timing and dosing optimization can significantly improve effectiveness without increasing total medication burden

- Side effect management strategies help maintain medication adherence while preserving quality of life

- Drug interactions and contraindications require careful monitoring, especially with multiple medications

- Pharmacists provide valuable expertise in medication optimization, compounding, and insurance navigation

Chapter 7: Supplement Strategies

Natural Mast Cell Support

The supplement aisle can feel like a maze of promising bottles and conflicting claims, each offering hope for better symptom control and improved quality of life. For people with MCAS, the appeal of natural approaches often stems from a desire to support healing without adding more synthetic medications to an already complex regimen. Yet navigating the world of supplements requires the same careful, evidence-based approach you use for prescription medications - perhaps even more so, given the less stringent regulation of dietary supplements.

Natural mast cell support through targeted supplementation can provide valuable benefits when used appropriately alongside conventional treatments. The key lies in understanding which supplements have solid research backing, how they work within your body's complex systems, and how to integrate them safely into your overall management plan. Your supplement strategy should complement, not replace, proven medical treatments while addressing nutritional gaps and supporting your body's natural healing processes.

Natural Mast Cell Stabilizers

Several natural compounds demonstrate mast cell stabilizing properties in research studies, offering potential benefits for MCAS patients seeking additional symptom control. These natural stabilizers work through various mechanisms to reduce mast cell degranulation and support overall immune system balance.

Quercetin stands out as one of the most well-researched natural mast cell stabilizers. This flavonoid, found in onions, apples, berries, and other colorful fruits and vegetables, has been shown to stabilize mast cell membranes and reduce histamine release. Research demonstrates that quercetin can inhibit mast cell activation triggered by various stimuli, making it a valuable addition to MCAS management protocols (15).

The effectiveness of quercetin often depends on absorption, which can be enhanced by taking it with bromelain, vitamin C, or other compounds that improve bioavailability. Most studies use doses ranging from 500-1000mg twice daily, though some patients benefit from higher amounts. Starting with lower doses and gradually increasing helps assess tolerance and optimal dosing for individual needs.

Luteolin represents another powerful flavonoid with mast cell stabilizing properties. Found in celery, parsley, and other green vegetables, luteolin has been shown to reduce both mast cell activation and the production of inflammatory cytokines. Some research suggests that luteolin may be even more potent than quercetin for certain types of mast cell stabilization.

Hesperidin and other citrus flavonoids provide additional mast cell stabilizing benefits. These compounds work synergistically with quercetin and luteolin to provide broader spectrum stabilization. Many patients find that combinations of flavonoids work better than single compounds alone.

Dr. Amanda, a naturopathic physician specializing in immune disorders, explains: "I often recommend starting with quercetin as the foundation of a natural mast cell stabilizing protocol. The research is strongest for quercetin, and most patients tolerate it well. We can then add other flavonoids based on individual response and specific symptom patterns."

Green tea extract contains epigallocatechin gallate (EGCG) and other polyphenols that demonstrate mast cell stabilizing properties. However, green tea extract requires careful consideration for MCAS patients since it can be stimulating and may not be well-tolerated by those sensitive to caffeine or tannins.

Dosing considerations for natural mast cell stabilizers often require higher amounts than typically found in multivitamins or general supplements. Therapeutic doses usually range from 500-2000mg daily for quercetin, though individual needs vary significantly. Taking these supplements with meals often improves tolerance and absorption.

Sarah, a 36-year-old graphic designer, found success with natural stabilizers: "I started taking quercetin and luteolin about six months ago, along with my prescription medications. I noticed that I had fewer minor reactions to everyday triggers - things like walking through the perfume section at the store didn't bother me as much. It's been a nice addition to my overall protocol."

Quality considerations become particularly important with natural mast cell stabilizers since supplement quality varies widely between manufacturers. Look for products that have been third-party tested for purity and potency. Standardized extracts often provide more consistent results than whole herb preparations.

Anti-Inflammatory Supplements

Chronic inflammation plays a significant role in MCAS symptom severity and overall health impact. Targeted anti-inflammatory supplements can help reduce overall inflammatory burden while supporting your body's natural healing processes and potentially reducing the frequency and severity of mast cell reactions.

Omega-3 fatty acids provide fundamental anti-inflammatory support through multiple mechanisms. EPA (eicosapentaenoic acid) and DHA (docosahexaenoic acid) from fish oil help produce specialized pro-resolving mediators that actively resolve inflammation rather than simply suppressing it. Research shows that adequate omega-3 intake can reduce inflammatory markers and support immune system balance (16).

The quality of omega-3 supplements varies significantly, with molecular distillation and third-party testing for contaminants being essential quality markers. Many MCAS patients find that they need higher doses than typically recommended - often 2-4 grams of combined EPA and DHA daily - to achieve anti-inflammatory benefits.

Curcumin offers potent anti-inflammatory effects through inhibition of multiple inflammatory pathways. The active compounds in turmeric have been extensively studied for their ability to reduce inflammatory cytokines and support immune system regulation. However, curcumin absorption is notoriously poor, requiring enhanced formulations or combination with piperine (black pepper extract) for optimal bioavailability.

Boswellia serrata extract provides anti-inflammatory benefits through inhibition of 5-lipoxygenase, an enzyme involved in leukotriene production. Since leukotrienes are important inflammatory mediators released by mast cells, boswellia may provide specific benefits for MCAS patients. Look for standardized extracts containing at least 65% boswellic acids.

Specialized pro-resolving mediators (SPMs) represent a newer category of supplements that support the active resolution of inflammation. These compounds, derived from omega-3 fatty acids, help the body complete the inflammatory process rather than leaving it in a chronic, unresolved state.

Dr. Robert, an integrative medicine physician, notes: "Many MCAS patients are stuck in chronic inflammatory states that perpetuate mast cell reactivity. Supporting inflammation resolution through targeted supplementation can help break this cycle and improve overall stability."

Dosing protocols for anti-inflammatory supplements often require consistent use over several months to see full benefits. Unlike symptom-relief supplements that may work quickly, anti-inflammatory support typically requires 8-12 weeks of consistent use to demonstrate significant effects.

Mark, a 43-year-old engineer, experienced gradual improvement: "I added high-quality fish oil and curcumin to my regimen about a year ago. The changes were subtle at first - maybe fewer aches and pains, better energy levels. But over several months, I realized I was having fewer overall flare-ups and seemed to recover more quickly from reactions when they did occur."

Interaction considerations require attention since some anti-inflammatory supplements can interact with medications, particularly blood thinners. Omega-3 fatty acids, curcumin, and boswellia can all affect blood clotting, requiring monitoring if you take anticoagulant medications.

Histamine-Degrading Supplements

Supporting your body's natural histamine metabolism can help reduce overall histamine burden and improve tolerance to histamine-containing foods and environmental exposures. Several supplements can enhance the activity of enzymes responsible for breaking down histamine.

Diamine oxidase (DAO) supplements provide direct enzyme support for histamine breakdown in the digestive system. DAO is the primary enzyme responsible for degrading dietary histamine, and some people have naturally low DAO activity or take medications that inhibit this enzyme. Supplemental DAO taken before meals can help break down dietary histamine before it causes symptoms.

The effectiveness of DAO supplements depends on timing and dosing. Taking DAO 15-20 minutes before meals allows the enzyme to be present in the digestive system when histamine-containing foods arrive. Most people need 10,000-20,000 HDU (histamine degrading units) per meal, though individual needs vary.

Vitamin B6 (pyridoxal-5-phosphate) serves as an essential cofactor for histamine metabolism. Adequate B6 levels are necessary for proper DAO function, and deficiency can worsen histamine intolerance. The active form of B6 (P5P) is often better absorbed and utilized than standard pyridoxine.

Vitamin C supports histamine metabolism through multiple pathways and can help stabilize mast cells. High-dose vitamin C (1-3 grams daily) may help reduce histamine levels and support overall immune function. However, some people are sensitive to certain forms of vitamin C, particularly synthetic ascorbic acid.

Copper is required for proper DAO enzyme function, and mild copper deficiency can contribute to histamine intolerance. However, copper supplementation requires careful monitoring since excess copper can cause oxidative stress and other health problems. Most people get adequate copper from food sources unless they have specific absorption issues.

Jennifer, a 38-year-old teacher, found DAO supplements helpful: "I started taking DAO enzymes before meals that contained higher histamine foods. It made a noticeable difference in my tolerance - I could eat small amounts of aged cheese or tomatoes without getting stomach cramps and flushing. It's not a cure-all, but it gives me more flexibility in my diet."

Timing strategies for histamine-degrading supplements require coordination with meals and other medications. DAO supplements work best when taken shortly before eating, while B6 and vitamin C can be taken with meals to improve absorption.

Quality considerations for enzyme supplements include stability and activity levels. DAO supplements should be stored properly and purchased from reputable manufacturers who test for enzyme activity. Some formulations include additional cofactors that may enhance effectiveness.

Gut Health and Microbiome Support

The digestive system plays a central role in MCAS for many patients, making gut health support a critical component of any supplement strategy. A healthy microbiome can help reduce inflammation, support immune function, and potentially reduce food sensitivities that trigger mast cell reactions.

Probiotics offer potential benefits for MCAS patients, though strain selection requires careful consideration. Some probiotic strains can produce histamine, potentially worsening symptoms in sensitive individuals. However, other strains can help break down histamine and support overall gut health.

Low-histamine probiotic strains include Lactobacillus rhamnosus, Lactobacillus plantarum, Bifidobacterium longum, and Bifidobacterium lactis. These strains are less likely to produce histamine and may help support healthy digestive function without triggering symptoms.

Prebiotic support helps feed beneficial bacteria and support microbiome diversity. However, many common prebiotics like inulin and FOS can cause digestive upset in sensitive individuals. Gentler options include partially hydrolyzed guar gum or specific resistant starches that are better tolerated.

Digestive enzymes can help improve food breakdown and reduce the likelihood of partially digested proteins triggering immune reactions. Broad-spectrum enzyme formulas that include proteases, lipases, and carbohydrases may help reduce digestive stress and improve nutrient absorption.

L-glutamine supports intestinal barrier function and may help reduce intestinal permeability that can contribute to food sensitivities. Doses of 5-15 grams daily are commonly used, though some people are sensitive to glutamine supplementation.

Dr. Lisa, a functional medicine practitioner, explains: "Gut health is fundamental for MCAS management, but we have to be careful about probiotic selection. I typically start with very small amounts of low-histamine strains and increase gradually while monitoring symptoms. Supporting gut barrier function with glutamine and gentle prebiotics often helps reduce overall reactivity."

Implementation strategies for gut health supplements require gradual introduction and careful monitoring. Start with single supplements rather than complex formulas to identify any that trigger symptoms. Many people need to introduce gut health supplements very slowly to avoid temporary worsening of symptoms.

Lisa, a 32-year-old nurse, improved her gut health gradually: "I tried probiotics several times before finding ones that worked for me. The key was starting with tiny amounts and increasing very slowly. I also focused on supporting my gut lining with glutamine and being very careful about prebiotic foods. It took about six months, but my digestive symptoms improved significantly."

Nervous System Support

The connection between the nervous system and mast cell activation makes nervous system support an important consideration for many MCAS patients. Supplements that support stress resilience, sleep quality, and nervous system function can help reduce the frequency and severity of stress-triggered reactions.

Magnesium provides fundamental support for nervous system function and stress resilience. Many people are deficient in magnesium, and deficiency can worsen anxiety, sleep problems, and stress reactivity. Different forms of magnesium have different properties - magnesium glycinate is often well-tolerated and promotes relaxation, while magnesium threonate may support cognitive function.

B-complex vitamins support nervous system function and stress resilience. B vitamins are often depleted during chronic stress and inflammation, making supplementation beneficial for many MCAS patients. However, some people are sensitive to certain forms of B vitamins, particularly folic acid and cyanocobalamin.

Adaptogens like ashwagandha, rhodiola, and holy basil can help support stress resilience and reduce cortisol dysregulation. These herbs work gradually over time to help the body adapt to stress more effectively. However, some people with autoimmune tendencies may not tolerate immune-stimulating adaptogens.

GABA and calming amino acids like glycine and taurine can help support relaxation and sleep quality. These supplements may be particularly helpful for patients who experience anxiety or sleep disturbances related to their MCAS symptoms.

Phosphatidylserine supports healthy cortisol rhythms and stress response. This phospholipid can help reduce excessive cortisol production and support better stress resilience over time.

Michael, a 45-year-old accountant, found nervous system support beneficial: "I started taking magnesium glycinate and a B-complex after noticing that stress was a major trigger for my reactions. The magnesium helped with my sleep quality, and I felt less reactive to everyday stressors. It didn't eliminate my MCAS symptoms, but it definitely helped me feel more resilient overall."

Sleep support considerations become particularly important since poor sleep can worsen mast cell stability. Natural sleep aids like melatonin, passionflower, or chamomile may help improve sleep quality without the side effects of prescription sleep medications. However, some people with MCAS are sensitive to herbal preparations.

Dosing timing for nervous system support supplements often works best when aligned with natural circadian rhythms. Magnesium and calming supplements typically work best when taken in the evening, while B vitamins are often better tolerated in the morning to avoid potential sleep disruption.

Quality and Safety Considerations

The supplement industry operates under different regulations than prescription medications, making quality and safety considerations particularly important for MCAS patients who may be sensitive to contaminants, fillers, or inconsistent potency.

Third-party testing provides independent verification of supplement purity and potency. Look for products that have been tested by organizations like NSF International, USP, or ConsumerLab. These certifications help ensure that products contain what they claim and are free from harmful contaminants.

Manufacturing standards vary widely between supplement companies. Look for companies that follow Good Manufacturing Practices (GMP) and have FDA-inspected facilities. Companies that voluntarily submit to additional quality standards often produce more reliable products.

Ingredient sensitivity requires careful attention to inactive ingredients that might trigger MCAS reactions. Common problematic ingredients include artificial colors, flavors, preservatives, and certain binding agents. Some people react to specific fillers like microcrystalline cellulose or magnesium stearate.

Allergen considerations become critical for people with multiple sensitivities. Many supplements are manufactured in facilities that also process common allergens like soy, dairy, or gluten. Cross-contamination can cause reactions in highly sensitive individuals.

Dr. Jennifer, a pharmacist specializing in integrative medicine, advises: "I always recommend that MCAS patients start with pharmaceutical-grade supplements from reputable companies. The few extra dollars spent on quality can prevent reactions from contaminants or inconsistent potency. It's also important to introduce supplements one at a time to identify any that cause problems."

Expiration dates and storage conditions affect supplement potency and safety. Many supplements lose potency over time, particularly those containing omega-3 fatty acids or probiotics. Store supplements in cool, dry conditions and replace them before expiration dates.

Interaction screening should include both prescription medications and other supplements. Some natural compounds can interact with medications or affect the absorption of other supplements. Keep detailed records of all supplements and medications to discuss with healthcare providers.

Timing and Interactions

Strategic timing of supplement intake can significantly affect their effectiveness and help minimize potential interactions with medications or other supplements. Understanding optimal timing helps you get the most benefit from your supplement regimen while avoiding complications.

Meal timing considerations affect absorption of many supplements. Fat-soluble vitamins (A, D, E, K) require dietary fat for optimal absorption and should be taken with meals containing some fat. Water-soluble vitamins like B vitamins and vitamin C can be taken with or without food, though some people tolerate them better with meals.

Medication spacing helps prevent interactions that could reduce effectiveness of either supplements or medications. Calcium and magnesium can interfere with the absorption of certain antibiotics and should be spaced several hours apart. Iron supplements can interfere with thyroid medications and should be taken at least four hours apart.

Supplement combinations can enhance or interfere with each other's effectiveness. Vitamin C enhances iron absorption but can reduce the effectiveness of certain B vitamins if taken in very high doses. Calcium and magnesium compete for absorption and may be better taken at different times of day.

Circadian timing optimizes supplements based on natural body rhythms. B vitamins often provide energy and are best taken in the morning, while magnesium and calming supplements work better in the evening. Melatonin should be taken 30-60 minutes before desired bedtime.

Sarah, a 41-year-old marketing manager, developed an effective timing system: "I take my B vitamins and vitamin C with breakfast, my quercetin and omega-3s with lunch, and my magnesium and probiotics with dinner. I space my iron supplement (taken three times per week) away from my other supplements and take it with vitamin C to improve absorption. It seems complicated, but it's become routine."

Strategic cycling may benefit some supplements, particularly those that can lose effectiveness with continuous use. Some practitioners recommend taking breaks from certain adaptogens or rotating different probiotic strains to maintain effectiveness.

Loading and maintenance phases apply to certain supplements that require higher initial doses to achieve therapeutic levels. Vitamin D often requires loading doses for people with deficiency, followed by lower maintenance doses. Omega-3 fatty acids may also benefit from higher initial doses.

Integrating Natural Support

Your supplement strategy should complement rather than replace proven medical treatments for MCAS. The goal is creating a synergistic approach where natural compounds enhance the effectiveness of your medical management while addressing nutritional gaps and supporting your body's healing processes.

The journey to finding your optimal supplement regimen requires the same systematic approach you use for other aspects of MCAS management. Start with foundational supplements that have strong research support, introduce new additions gradually, and monitor your response carefully. Not every supplement that helps others will work for you, and your needs may change as your overall health improves.

Quality becomes paramount when dealing with a sensitive immune system that may react to contaminants or inconsistent formulations. Investing in high-quality supplements from reputable manufacturers helps ensure that you're getting therapeutic benefits rather than creating new problems. The partnership between natural and conventional approaches often provides the most stable and sustainable symptom management over time.

Key Learning Points

- Natural mast cell stabilizers like quercetin and luteolin provide research-backed support for reducing mast cell activation

- Anti-inflammatory supplements including omega-3 fatty acids and curcumin help address chronic inflammation that perpetuates MCAS symptoms

- Histamine-degrading supplements such as DAO enzymes and vitamin B6 support the body's natural histamine breakdown processes

- Gut health and microbiome support require careful probiotic strain selection and gradual implementation to avoid triggering symptoms

- Nervous system support through magnesium, B vitamins, and adaptogens can help reduce stress-triggered mast cell reactions

- Quality and safety considerations are critical due to variable supplement regulation and potential sensitivity to contaminants

- Strategic timing and interaction awareness optimize supplement effectiveness while preventing interference with medications

Chapter 8: Exercise and Movement Adaptation

- Staying Active with MCAS

The irony strikes you as you lace up your sneakers for what should be a simple walk around the block. The same body that desperately needs movement for health and stress relief may rebel against the very activity designed to help it. Exercise-induced reactions can transform what was once a source of joy and vitality into a source of anxiety and unpredictable symptoms. Yet movement remains one of the most powerful tools for supporting overall health, managing stress, and maintaining quality of life with MCAS.

The relationship between exercise and mast cell activation is complex and highly individual. Some people find that gentle movement helps stabilize their symptoms, while others discover that certain types of exercise consistently trigger reactions. Understanding this relationship allows you to harness the benefits of physical activity while avoiding the pitfalls that can worsen your condition. The goal isn't to avoid movement entirely, but to find the sweet spot where exercise supports rather than undermines your health.

Exercise and Mast Cell Activation

Physical activity can trigger mast cell activation through multiple pathways, making it essential to understand these mechanisms before developing your personal exercise strategy. The triggers range from obvious physical stressors to subtle changes in body chemistry that occur during different types of movement.

Heat generation during exercise represents one of the most common triggers for exercise-induced reactions. As your body temperature rises, blood vessels dilate and circulation increases, which can activate temperature-sensitive mast cells. This mechanism explains why some people experience flushing, hives, or cardiovascular symptoms during or after exercise, particularly in warm environments.

Mechanical stimulation from repetitive movement, vibration, or pressure can directly activate mast cells in affected tissues. Running may trigger reactions in people with pressure-sensitive mast cells in their feet, while swimming might affect those sensitive to water pressure or temperature changes. Contact sports or activities involving equipment pressure can cause localized reactions in sensitive areas.

Increased circulation during exercise enhances the distribution of any circulating triggers throughout your body. If you've been exposed to dietary histamine, environmental chemicals, or other triggers before exercising, the increased blood flow can amplify your reaction to these substances.

Dehydration and electrolyte changes that occur during prolonged or intense exercise can affect mast cell stability. Dehydration concentrates any circulating mediators while electrolyte imbalances can alter cellular function. Some people find they're more reactive to exercise when they're not properly hydrated or when their sodium levels are low.

Dr. Michael, a sports medicine physician who treats several MCAS patients, explains: "Exercise-induced mast cell reactions often involve multiple triggers acting together. A patient might tolerate moderate exercise in cool weather but react strongly to the same activity on a hot day or when they're stressed. Understanding these interactions helps develop safer exercise protocols."

Stress hormone release during intense exercise can directly trigger mast cell activation in some individuals. The adrenaline and cortisol released during high-intensity activity may activate stress-sensitive mast cells, leading to symptoms that can be mistaken for normal exercise responses.

Exercise-induced anaphylaxis represents the most severe form of exercise-related mast cell activation. This condition can be triggered by exercise alone or by the combination of exercise with specific foods, medications, or environmental exposures. Symptoms can include widespread hives, difficulty breathing, gastrointestinal distress, and cardiovascular collapse.

Jennifer, a 34-year-old marketing manager, experienced exercise-induced reactions: "I loved running before my MCAS diagnosis, but I started having episodes where I'd get severe flushing and nausea during my runs. It took several episodes before I realized the pattern - it was worse on hot days or when I'd eaten certain foods before running. Learning to modify my routine let me get back to the activity I enjoyed."

Delayed reactions can occur hours after exercise, making the connection between activity and symptoms less obvious. Some people feel fine during exercise but develop symptoms 2-4 hours later as inflammatory mediators continue circulating through their system.

Safe Exercise Guidelines

Developing safe exercise practices requires a systematic approach that prioritizes symptom prevention while maintaining the health benefits of physical activity. These guidelines provide a framework for staying active while minimizing the risk of exercise-induced reactions.

Start slowly and progress gradually regardless of your previous fitness level. MCAS can change your exercise tolerance significantly, and what you could do before your diagnosis may no longer be appropriate. Begin with very gentle activities and increase intensity, duration, or frequency only as your body demonstrates consistent tolerance.

Monitor your baseline stability before beginning any exercise session. If you're already experiencing symptoms, having a stressful day, or dealing with other triggers, consider modifying or postponing your planned activity. Exercise when your mast cells are already activated can amplify reactions significantly.

Temperature management becomes critical for preventing heat-induced reactions. Exercise in cool environments when possible, use cooling strategies like cold towels or ice packs, and avoid outdoor activities during peak heat hours. Indoor activities with good air conditioning often work better than outdoor exercise during summer months.

Hydration strategies should begin before you start exercising and continue throughout your activity. Drink water steadily rather than waiting until you feel thirsty. Some people benefit from electrolyte replacement, particularly if they're taking medications that affect fluid balance or if they sweat heavily.

Pre-exercise medication timing can help prevent reactions in people who consistently experience exercise-induced symptoms. Taking antihistamines 30-60 minutes before exercise may provide protective benefits. Some people benefit from using mast cell stabilizers before anticipated trigger activities.

Sarah, a 41-year-old teacher, developed effective safety protocols: "I learned to check my symptom level before exercising and have a scale from 1-10. If I'm above a 5, I do gentle stretching instead of my planned workout. I always exercise indoors with air conditioning, keep water nearby, and take my antihistamines an hour before more intense activities."

Environmental considerations extend beyond temperature to include air quality, allergen exposure, and chemical triggers. Avoid exercising outdoors on high pollution days or during peak pollen seasons if these affect you. Choose facilities with good ventilation and minimal use of strong cleaning chemicals or air fresheners.

Duration and intensity limits help prevent the cumulative effects that can trigger reactions. Many people with MCAS find they have a threshold for exercise intensity or duration beyond which they consistently react. Identify your personal limits and respect them, even on days when you feel you could push harder.

Adapting Different Types of Exercise

Different forms of exercise pose varying risks and benefits for people with MCAS. Understanding how to modify activities allows you to participate safely in a wide range of physical activities while managing your specific triggers and limitations.

Cardiovascular exercise provides important health benefits but requires careful modification for many MCAS patients. Walking represents the safest starting point for most people, allowing gradual conditioning while monitoring for reactions. Treadmill walking in climate-controlled environments often works better than outdoor walking for temperature-sensitive individuals.

Swimming can be excellent for MCAS patients since the water provides natural cooling and supports body weight, reducing mechanical stress. However, pool chemicals, temperature variations, or pressure changes can trigger some people. Start with short sessions in well-maintained pools with comfortable water temperatures.

Strength training allows for controlled progression and can be easily modified based on daily tolerance. Resistance bands, light weights, or bodyweight exercises can provide muscle strengthening without the cardiovascular stress of aerobic activities. Focus on proper form and gradual progression rather than lifting heavy weights.

Flexibility and mobility work often represents the safest form of exercise for MCAS patients. Gentle stretching, yoga, or tai chi can provide movement benefits while promoting relaxation and stress reduction. These activities typically generate less heat and place less stress on the cardiovascular system.

Mark, a 38-year-old engineer, found success with adapted strength training: "I had to give up my intense gym workouts, but I discovered that resistance band exercises at home worked really well for me. I could control the temperature, take breaks when needed, and gradually increase resistance as my tolerance improved. It's different from what I used to do, but it keeps me strong without triggering reactions."

High-intensity activities like running, cycling, or team sports may need significant modification or avoidance, particularly during the initial phases of MCAS management. Some people can return to these activities once their condition is well-controlled, while others find that lower-intensity alternatives work better long-term.

Group fitness classes require careful evaluation of the environment, instructor awareness, and your ability to modify activities as needed. Choose instructors who understand medical limitations and classes that allow for individual modifications. Avoid classes in overheated rooms or those with strong music or lighting that might trigger sensitivities.

Pre and Post-Exercise Protocols

Developing consistent pre and post-exercise routines helps optimize your body's response to physical activity while minimizing the risk of reactions. These protocols become particularly important for people who experience delayed or cumulative effects from exercise.

Pre-exercise preparation begins hours before your planned activity. Ensure adequate hydration starting the day before intensive exercise. Avoid known trigger foods for several hours before exercising, as the combination of triggers plus exercise can amplify reactions. Consider timing your exercise around your most stable periods of the day.

Medication timing may need adjustment around exercise sessions. Some people benefit from taking antihistamines before exercise, while others find that certain medications affect their exercise tolerance. Work with your healthcare provider to optimize medication timing around your activity schedule.

Warm-up protocols should be gradual and gentle, allowing your body to adjust slowly to increased activity. Start with very light movement and gradually increase intensity over 10-15 minutes. Monitor for early warning signs like flushing, increased heart rate beyond normal exercise responses, or gastrointestinal symptoms.

Environmental setup includes ensuring comfortable temperature, good ventilation, and easy access to water and emergency medications. Have cooling strategies available like fans, cold towels, or ice packs. Keep your rescue medications easily accessible during all exercise sessions.

Lisa, a 35-year-old nurse, developed a thorough pre-exercise routine: "I start hydrating the night before planned exercise and avoid my trigger foods after lunch if I'm exercising the next morning. I take my antihistamines with breakfast, set up fans in my exercise area, and always have my rescue inhaler and extra antihistamines nearby. The preparation takes time, but it's prevented many reactions."

Post-exercise protocols focus on supporting recovery while monitoring for delayed reactions. Continue hydrating immediately after exercise and monitor your temperature for several hours. Some people benefit from cooling strategies like cool showers or cold packs applied to pulse points.

Recovery monitoring should continue for 4-6 hours after exercise since delayed reactions can occur as inflammatory mediators continue circulating. Track symptoms like fatigue, mood changes, digestive issues, or skin reactions that might appear hours after your workout.

Managing Exercise Limitations

Accepting and working within your exercise limitations requires a shift in mindset from "what I used to do" to "what serves my body now." This transition can be challenging, particularly for people who were very active before developing MCAS, but it opens the door to finding new forms of movement that support rather than stress your system.

Redefining fitness goals means focusing on consistency and symptom management rather than performance metrics. Success might be measured by how consistently you can maintain an activity routine without triggering reactions rather than how fast you can run or how much weight you can lift.

Variable tolerance patterns require flexible planning since your exercise tolerance may change from day to day based on overall mast cell stability, stress levels, weather conditions, or other factors. Develop multiple exercise options at different intensity levels so you can choose activities that match your daily capacity.

Energy management becomes crucial since exercise should energize rather than deplete you. Many MCAS patients have limited energy reserves, making it important to choose activities that provide benefits without exhausting your daily energy budget. Gentle movement often provides more sustainable benefits than intense exercise.

Social considerations may require adjusting group activities or explaining limitations to exercise partners. Some people find it helpful to exercise alone initially while learning their limits, then gradually return to social activities as their tolerance improves.

Dr. Jennifer, a rehabilitation specialist, notes: "I often see MCAS patients who are frustrated because they can't do what they used to do. The key is helping them find activities they can do consistently. A daily 15-minute walk that doesn't trigger symptoms is far more beneficial than weekend warrior activities that cause reactions."

Symptom tracking helps identify patterns in your exercise tolerance and optimal timing for different activities. Keep records of activities, environmental conditions, pre-exercise symptom levels, and post-exercise responses to identify what works best for your body.

Alternative movement strategies can provide many of the benefits of traditional exercise while being gentler on reactive systems. Chair exercises for those with severe limitations, water therapy, gentle dance, or even household activities can contribute to your overall movement goals.

Building Fitness Gradually

The process of rebuilding or maintaining fitness with MCAS requires patience and a long-term perspective. Progress may be slower than you'd like, but consistent gentle activity often provides better long-term benefits than sporadic intense exercise that triggers reactions.

Baseline assessment helps establish your current tolerance and provides a starting point for gradual progression. This might involve timing how long you can walk without symptoms, noting which activities trigger reactions, and identifying optimal environmental conditions for exercise.

Progressive overload principles still apply but must be modified for MCAS. Instead of increasing intensity weekly, you might increase duration by just a few minutes monthly or add resistance only after several weeks of consistent tolerance. The progression should be so gradual that it doesn't stress your system.

Consistency over intensity becomes the guiding principle for MCAS fitness development. Regular gentle activity provides more benefit than occasional intense sessions. Aim for activities you can perform daily or every other day rather than sporadic challenging workouts.

Plateau acceptance recognizes that your fitness progression may level off at points that feel frustrating but represent your body's current capacity. These plateaus aren't failures - they're information about your current limits and opportunities to maintain your achieved level while continuing other aspects of MCAS management.

Michael, a 42-year-old accountant, describes his gradual progression: "I started with five-minute walks around my block because that's all I could tolerate without getting flushed and dizzy. It took six months to work up to 20-minute walks, but now I can walk consistently without reactions. It's not the five-mile runs I used to do, but it's sustainable movement that makes me feel better."

Seasonal adjustments may be necessary as your tolerance changes with weather, daylight, and other environmental factors. Many people find they can do more intense activities in cooler months while needing to scale back during summer heat or high-allergen seasons.

Cross-training approaches help prevent overuse of specific muscle groups while providing variety in your routine. Alternate between different types of gentle activities to maintain interest and work different aspects of fitness without overstressing any single system.

Activity Modification Strategies

Learning to modify activities allows you to participate in many forms of movement while respecting your body's limitations. These adaptations often require creativity but can help maintain quality of life and social connections around physical activities.

Intensity reduction represents the most straightforward modification strategy. Lower the intensity of any activity until it falls within your tolerance zone. This might mean walking instead of jogging, using lighter weights, or taking more frequent rest breaks during activities.

Duration adjustments allow participation in activities that might be problematic at full length. Attend part of a fitness class, play sports for shorter periods, or break longer activities into smaller segments with rest periods.

Environmental modifications can make previously problematic activities tolerable. Exercise indoors instead of outdoors, use fans or air conditioning, choose cooler times of day, or select locations with better air quality or fewer trigger exposures.

Equipment adaptations help reduce physical stress while maintaining activity benefits. Use supportive shoes for walking, wear cooling vests during exercise, or choose low-impact equipment that reduces joint stress while providing cardiovascular benefits.

Sarah, a 36-year-old graphic designer, adapted her yoga practice: "I loved hot yoga before MCAS, but the heat became a major trigger. I found a gentle yoga class in a normally-heated room and learned to modify poses that caused flushing. I use a small fan during practice and choose spots near the door for fresh air. It's different from my old practice, but it still provides the stress relief and flexibility I need."

Timing strategies can significantly affect exercise tolerance. Many people have optimal times of day for physical activity based on their medication schedules, symptom patterns, or energy levels. Experiment with different timing to find your most stable periods for movement.

Social modifications help maintain exercise-based social connections while respecting your limitations. Meet friends for gentle walks instead of intense hikes, suggest indoor activities during extreme weather, or participate in group activities at your own pace while others continue at higher intensities.

Movement as Medicine

Exercise for people with MCAS requires a fundamental shift in perspective from performance to self-care, from pushing limits to respecting boundaries, and from comparing to others to honoring your own body's needs. This shift isn't a limitation - it's a more sophisticated understanding of how to use movement as medicine rather than as a test of willpower or endurance.

The goal isn't to return to your pre-MCAS activity level, though some people do achieve this over time. The goal is to find sustainable ways to move your body that support your overall health without triggering the very symptoms you're working to manage. This approach often leads to a more mindful, intuitive relationship with physical activity that serves you better in the long run.

Your exercise journey with MCAS will be unique to your triggers, limitations, and preferences. What matters is finding forms of movement that you can maintain consistently while feeling good in your body. The activities that serve you best may change over time as your condition stabilizes or as your life circumstances shift, and that flexibility becomes part of your long-term success strategy.

Key Learning Points

- Exercise can trigger mast cell activation through heat generation, mechanical stimulation, and stress hormone release

- Safe exercise guidelines include gradual progression, temperature management, and careful hydration strategies

- Different types of exercise require specific adaptations based on individual triggers and tolerance levels

- Pre and post-exercise protocols help optimize safety and monitor for delayed reactions

- Exercise limitations require redefining fitness goals and accepting variable tolerance patterns

- Building fitness gradually with consistency over intensity provides sustainable long-term benefits

- Activity modification strategies allow participation in preferred activities while respecting physical limitations

Chapter 9: Stress Management and Nervous System Support

- Calming Your Body and Mind

The moment you feel stress building - that familiar tightness in your chest, the racing thoughts, the growing sense of urgency - your body prepares for what it perceives as threat. But when you have MCAS, this natural stress response can quickly cascade into physical symptoms that extend far beyond normal stress reactions. Your heart rate might spike beyond typical stress levels, your skin might flush or break out in hives, or your digestive system might revolt in ways that leave you feeling helpless and frustrated.

Understanding the intimate connection between stress and mast cell activation opens doorways to powerful management strategies that address both your emotional well-being and your physical symptoms. The nervous system and immune system communicate constantly, and learning to support this communication can significantly improve your daily symptom control and overall quality of life. Stress management for MCAS isn't just about feeling calmer - it's about preventing stress from triggering the very symptoms that create more stress.

The Stress-Mast Cell Connection

The relationship between psychological stress and mast cell activation involves complex biological pathways that directly link your emotional state to your physical symptoms. Understanding these connections helps explain why stress management becomes such a powerful tool for MCAS control and why emotional triggers can cause very real physical reactions.

The hypothalamic-pituitary-adrenal (HPA) axis serves as the primary stress response system, releasing hormones like cortisol and adrenaline when you perceive threat or pressure. These stress hormones can directly activate mast cells, particularly in people with already sensitive systems. Chronic stress keeps this system activated, creating a state where mast cells remain on high alert (17).

Corticotropin-releasing hormone (CRH) represents one of the most direct connections between stress and mast cell activation. Released by the brain during stress, CRH can directly bind to mast cell receptors and trigger degranulation. This explains why emotional stress can cause immediate physical symptoms in many MCAS patients.

Sympathetic nervous system activation during stress releases norepinephrine and epinephrine, which can activate mast cells throughout the body. This system controls the "fight or flight" response, and in people with MCAS, it can trigger symptoms like flushing, heart palpitations, and digestive upset even when the stressor is purely psychological.

Inflammatory feedback loops create a cycle where stress triggers mast cell activation, which releases inflammatory mediators, which can worsen mood and stress levels, leading to further mast cell activation. Breaking this cycle requires addressing both the stress response and the physical inflammation.

Dr. Rachel, a psychiatrist specializing in medical stress management, explains: "Many MCAS patients feel like they're going crazy because emotional stress causes very real physical symptoms. Understanding that this connection is biological, not psychological, helps patients develop effective coping strategies without self-blame."

Chronic stress effects differ from acute stress in their impact on mast cell stability. While short-term stress might cause temporary symptoms, chronic stress can lead to persistent mast cell activation, increased trigger sensitivity, and worsening of baseline symptoms. This makes ongoing stress management essential rather than optional.

Individual stress vulnerability varies significantly between people with MCAS. Some people are highly stress-reactive, while others can tolerate significant psychological pressure without physical symptoms. Identifying your personal stress triggers and early warning signs helps you intervene before stress escalates into physical reactions.

Jennifer, a 39-year-old project manager, discovered her stress-symptom connection: "I thought I was handling work stress pretty well until I started tracking my symptoms alongside my stress levels. I realized that my worst MCAS days consistently followed high-stress periods at work. Once I saw the pattern, I could start addressing the stress before it triggered physical symptoms."

Sleep and stress interactions create additional complexity since poor sleep worsens stress tolerance while stress disrupts sleep quality. This creates another feedback loop that can destabilize mast cell function and worsen overall symptom control.

Nervous System Dysregulation in MCAS

Many people with MCAS experience nervous system dysregulation that goes beyond typical stress responses. This dysregulation can affect everything from heart rate and blood pressure to temperature regulation and digestive function, making nervous system support a critical component of comprehensive MCAS management.

Autonomic nervous system dysfunction commonly occurs in MCAS patients, affecting the automatic functions that regulate heart rate, blood pressure, digestion, and temperature control. This dysfunction can manifest as postural orthostatic tachycardia syndrome (POTS), gastroparesis, temperature intolerance, or other symptoms that seem unrelated to stress but actually reflect nervous system imbalance.

Sympathetic dominance occurs when the "fight or flight" branch of the nervous system becomes overactive relative to the "rest and digest" parasympathetic system. This imbalance can contribute to chronic anxiety, sleep problems, digestive issues, and increased mast cell reactivity. Many MCAS patients benefit from interventions that support parasympathetic activation.

Hypervigilance represents a state where the nervous system remains on high alert, scanning for potential threats even in safe environments. This constant state of alertness can be exhausting and can lower the threshold for mast cell activation. People with hypervigilance often feel "wired but tired" and have difficulty relaxing even when they want to.

Sensory processing changes can occur when nervous system dysregulation affects how you process sensory information. Sounds may seem louder, lights brighter, or touch more intense than before. These sensory sensitivities can become triggers for mast cell activation, creating additional stress and symptom complexity.

Dr. Michael, a neurologist familiar with MCAS, notes: "Nervous system dysregulation in MCAS isn't just about anxiety or depression - it's about fundamental changes in how the nervous system processes information and regulates body functions. Addressing this dysregulation often improves both neurological and immune symptoms."

Cognitive effects of nervous system dysregulation include brain fog, difficulty concentrating, memory problems, and decision-making challenges. These cognitive symptoms can create stress and frustration, which then worsen the nervous system dysfunction. Supporting cognitive function often requires addressing the underlying nervous system imbalance.

Emotional regulation challenges may develop when nervous system dysregulation affects mood stability. You might find yourself more emotionally reactive than usual, with stronger responses to situations that previously wouldn't have bothered you. This increased emotional reactivity can trigger mast cell activation and physical symptoms.

Stress Reduction Techniques

Effective stress reduction for MCAS requires techniques that address both the immediate stress response and the underlying nervous system dysregulation. The most effective approaches typically combine multiple techniques to provide comprehensive support for stress resilience and nervous system balance.

Progressive muscle relaxation teaches you to systematically tense and release different muscle groups, helping you recognize and release physical tension that accumulates during stress. This technique can be particularly helpful for MCAS patients who carry stress in their bodies and may not realize how much physical tension they're holding.

Start with your feet and work upward through your body, tensing each muscle group for 5-10 seconds before releasing and focusing on the sensation of relaxation. Many people find guided recordings helpful when learning this technique. Practice when you're not stressed so the relaxation response becomes automatic and available during challenging times.

Deep breathing exercises activate the parasympathetic nervous system and can quickly shift your body from stress mode to relaxation mode. The key is breathing slowly and deeply, focusing on making your exhale longer than your inhale to maximize the calming response.

The 4-7-8 breathing pattern works well for many people: breathe in for 4 counts, hold for 7 counts, exhale for 8 counts. Repeat this cycle 4-6 times. Box breathing (4 counts in, 4 counts hold, 4 counts out, 4 counts hold) provides another effective pattern that's easy to remember during stressful situations.

Grounding techniques help you return to the present moment when stress, anxiety, or overwhelm threaten to spiral out of control. The 5-4-3-2-1 technique involves identifying 5 things you can see, 4 things you can touch, 3 things you can hear, 2 things you can smell, and 1 thing you can taste. This engages your sensory system and interrupts stress spirals.

Sarah, a 34-year-old teacher, uses grounding during MCAS flares: "When I feel a reaction starting and I know stress is making it worse, I do the 5-4-3-2-1 technique. It helps me stay calm instead of panicking, which often prevents the reaction from getting as severe. Sometimes just staying calm is enough to keep symptoms manageable."

Visualization techniques can create mental refuge and activate relaxation responses even when you can't physically remove yourself from stressful situations. Develop detailed mental images of places where you feel completely safe and calm - perhaps a beach, forest, or cozy room. Practice visiting this mental space regularly so it becomes easily accessible during stress.

Cognitive reframing helps you change how you think about stressful situations, often reducing their emotional impact. Instead of thinking "This is terrible and I can't handle it," try "This is challenging, but I have tools to manage it" or "This feeling will pass." This isn't about positive thinking - it's about developing more balanced, realistic perspectives.

Mindfulness and Meditation

Mindfulness practices offer powerful tools for managing both stress and MCAS symptoms by teaching you to observe your thoughts, emotions, and physical sensations without becoming overwhelmed by them. Regular mindfulness practice can reduce baseline stress levels while improving your ability to respond rather than react to challenging situations.

Mindfulness basics involve paying attention to the present moment without judgment. This means noticing what's happening in your mind and body right now without trying to change it or getting caught up in stories about what it means. For MCAS patients, this can be particularly helpful in observing symptoms without the additional stress of fighting or fearing them.

Body scan meditation involves systematically focusing attention on different parts of your body, noticing sensations without trying to change them. This practice can help you develop better awareness of physical tension, early warning signs of reactions, and the difference between symptoms and anxiety about symptoms.

Start with just 5-10 minutes of body scan practice, gradually working up to longer sessions as your attention span improves. Many people find guided body scan recordings helpful when starting this practice. The goal isn't to feel different - it's to notice what you're already feeling with greater clarity and less reactivity.

Mindful breathing uses the breath as an anchor for attention, helping you develop concentration while activating the parasympathetic nervous system. You don't need to change your breathing - just notice the natural rhythm of inhalation and exhalation. When your mind wanders (which it will), gently return attention to the breath without self-judgment.

Walking meditation combines gentle movement with mindfulness practice, which can be ideal for MCAS patients who find sitting meditation challenging. Walk slowly and deliberately, paying attention to the sensations of your feet touching the ground, the movement of your legs, and the rhythm of your steps.

Mark, a 41-year-old engineer, found mindfulness transformative: "I was skeptical about meditation, but my doctor suggested it for stress management. I started with just five minutes of breathing meditation daily. After a few months, I noticed I was less reactive to small stressors and could catch myself before stress spiraled into physical symptoms."

Loving-kindness meditation can be particularly helpful for MCAS patients who struggle with self-criticism or frustration about their symptoms. This practice involves directing well-wishes toward yourself and others, starting with phrases like "May I be happy, may I be healthy, may I be at peace." Extending compassion to yourself can reduce the stress of self-judgment.

Informal mindfulness involves bringing mindful attention to daily activities like eating, washing dishes, or walking. This helps you develop the skill of present-moment awareness without requiring additional time for formal meditation practice.

Breathing Techniques

Breathing represents one of the most immediate and powerful tools for managing stress and supporting nervous system regulation. Unlike other stress management techniques that require learning and practice, breathing is always available and can provide rapid relief when stress threatens to trigger physical symptoms.

Diaphragmatic breathing activates the parasympathetic nervous system more effectively than shallow chest breathing. Place one hand on your chest and one on your belly. Breathe so that the hand on your belly moves more than the hand on your chest. This deeper breathing pattern signals safety to your nervous system.

Practice diaphragmatic breathing when you're calm so it becomes natural and available during stressful moments. Many people find it helpful to practice for 5-10 minutes twice daily until the pattern becomes automatic.

Extended exhale breathing specifically activates the parasympathetic nervous system by making your exhale longer than your inhale. Try breathing in for 4 counts and out for 6-8 counts, adjusting the timing to what feels comfortable for you. The longer exhale signals to your nervous system that you're safe and can relax.

Coherent breathing involves breathing at a rate of about 5 breaths per minute, which optimizes heart rate variability and nervous system balance. Breathe in for 6 counts and out for 6 counts, maintaining this rhythm for 5-10 minutes. This practice can help synchronize your cardiovascular and nervous systems.

Breath awareness simply involves noticing your natural breathing without trying to change it. This practice can help you recognize how stress affects your breathing patterns and develop greater awareness of your internal state. Many people discover they hold their breath during stress without realizing it.

Lisa, a 37-year-old nurse, uses breathing for reaction management: "When I feel an MCAS reaction starting, I immediately start doing extended exhale breathing. It doesn't stop the reaction, but it often keeps it from getting as severe and helps me stay calm enough to take my rescue medications if needed."

Humming breath involves making a humming sound on the exhale, which creates vibrations that can be particularly calming for the nervous system. This technique also naturally extends the exhale and can provide both physical and emotional soothing during stress.

Box breathing provides a structured pattern that can be helpful during acute stress or panic. Breathe in for 4 counts, hold for 4 counts, exhale for 4 counts, hold for 4 counts. Repeat this cycle 4-6 times or until you feel your nervous system settling.

Progressive Muscle Relaxation

Progressive muscle relaxation (PMR) teaches you to systematically tense and release different muscle groups, helping you develop awareness of physical tension while learning to activate the relaxation response. This technique can be particularly beneficial for MCAS patients who carry stress in their bodies or who experience muscle tension as part of their symptom complex.

Basic PMR technique involves tensing specific muscle groups for 5-10 seconds, then releasing the tension while focusing on the sensation of relaxation for 15-20 seconds before moving to the next muscle group. Start with your feet and work systematically up through your body, ending with your face and scalp.

Muscle group progression typically follows this pattern: right foot and calf, left foot and calf, right thigh and buttock, left thigh and buttock, abdomen, right hand and forearm, left hand and forearm, right upper arm, left upper arm, shoulders, neck, face, and scalp. Adjust this sequence based on your comfort and any areas of particular tension.

Tension levels should be firm enough to notice the contrast when you release, but not so intense that you cause pain or strain. About 70% of maximum tension usually works well. People with muscle pain or injury may need to use very light tension or focus primarily on the relaxation phase.

Release and relaxation phases require equal attention to the tension phases. After releasing muscle tension, spend time noticing the sensations of relaxation - warmth, heaviness, softness, or whatever you experience. This helps train your nervous system to recognize and recreate the relaxed state.

Jennifer, a 33-year-old accountant, found PMR helpful for sleep: "I was having trouble falling asleep because my mind would race and my body felt tense from the day's stress. Doing progressive muscle relaxation in bed helps me physically let go of the day and signals to my body that it's time to rest. It's made a huge difference in my sleep quality."

Modified PMR can be adapted for people with physical limitations or those who find full-body tension uncomfortable. You can focus on just a few muscle groups, use lighter tension, or even practice "release-only" versions where you simply focus on letting go of existing tension without adding more.

Daily applications of PMR can include using mini-versions throughout the day, such as tensing and releasing your shoulders during work stress or doing quick hand and arm exercises when you notice tension building. These abbreviated versions help you apply the relaxation skills in real-time situations.

Cognitive Behavioral Strategies

Cognitive behavioral approaches help you identify and change thought patterns that increase stress and potentially trigger mast cell reactions. These strategies focus on the relationship between thoughts, emotions, and physical symptoms, providing tools for breaking cycles that worsen both stress and MCAS symptoms.

Thought awareness forms the foundation of cognitive behavioral work. Many people aren't fully aware of their automatic thoughts, especially those that increase stress and anxiety. Start by noticing thoughts that arise during stressful situations or when MCAS symptoms occur. Common patterns include catastrophizing, all-or-nothing thinking, and assuming the worst possible outcomes.

Cognitive distortions represent common thinking patterns that increase stress unnecessarily. These include catastrophizing ("This reaction means something terrible is happening"), fortune telling ("I know I'm going to have a bad reaction"), mind reading ("Everyone thinks I'm making this up"), and all-or-nothing thinking ("If I can't do everything perfectly, I'm a failure").

Thought challenging involves questioning automatic thoughts and developing more balanced, realistic alternatives.Ask yourself: "Is this thought helpful? Is it accurate? What evidence do I have for and against this thought? What would I tell a friend in this situation?" This process helps you develop more balanced perspectives that reduce stress.

Behavioral experiments test the accuracy of anxiety-provoking thoughts through carefully planned activities. If you believe that any stress will cause a severe MCAS reaction, you might gradually expose yourself to manageable stressors while monitoring your actual symptoms. Often, you'll discover that your fear is worse than the reality.

Activity scheduling helps combat the tendency to avoid activities due to fear of triggering symptoms. Schedule pleasant, meaningful activities even when you don't feel like doing them. This prevents the downward spiral of isolation and inactivity that can worsen both mood and physical symptoms.

Michael, a 44-year-old teacher, used cognitive strategies effectively: "I realized I was constantly predicting disaster - thinking every small symptom meant I was heading for a major reaction. Learning to question these thoughts and look for evidence helped me stay calmer, which actually reduced my reaction frequency. My thoughts were making my symptoms worse."

Problem-solving techniques help address actual stressors rather than just managing your response to them. Break large problems into smaller, manageable steps. Focus on what you can control rather than what you can't. Develop action plans for common stressful situations so you feel more prepared and less overwhelmed.

Acceptance strategies help you cope with aspects of MCAS that you can't change or control. This doesn't mean passive resignation - it means acknowledging reality so you can focus your energy on effective responses rather than fighting unchangeable circumstances.

Building Resilience

Resilience represents your ability to adapt to stress, recover from challenges, and maintain emotional stability despite ongoing health concerns. Building resilience helps you manage both the daily stresses of life and the specific challenges of living with MCAS more effectively.

Stress inoculation involves gradually exposing yourself to manageable stressors while practicing coping skills, similar to how vaccines work by exposing you to small amounts of a threat. Start with minor stressors and practice your stress management techniques, gradually building confidence in your ability to handle larger challenges.

Social support systems provide crucial buffering against stress and help you maintain perspective during difficult times. Cultivate relationships with people who understand your condition and can provide both emotional support and practical assistance. This might include family, friends, support groups, or healthcare providers.

Meaning-making helps you find purpose and significance even in the midst of health challenges. This might involve identifying how your MCAS experience has taught you valuable lessons, connected you with others, or motivated you to help people facing similar challenges. Finding meaning in suffering can significantly reduce its psychological impact.

Self-compassion involves treating yourself with the same kindness you would offer a good friend facing similar challenges. Many people with chronic health conditions are incredibly hard on themselves, which adds stress and worsens symptoms. Practice speaking to yourself with understanding and patience rather than criticism and judgment.

Dr. Sarah, a psychologist specializing in chronic illness, explains: "Resilience isn't about being tough or never feeling stressed. It's about developing skills and perspectives that help you bounce back from difficulties more quickly and completely. For MCAS patients, resilience can literally reduce symptom severity by decreasing stress-related triggers."

Flexibility and adaptability help you adjust your expectations and approaches when circumstances change. MCAS symptoms can be unpredictable, requiring flexibility in plans and goals. Developing comfort with uncertainty and change reduces the stress of trying to control uncontrollable factors.

Resource development involves building a toolkit of coping strategies, support systems, and practical resources that you can draw upon during challenging times. This might include stress management techniques, emergency action plans, supportive relationships, financial resources, or spiritual practices.

Sarah, a 38-year-old marketing manager, describes her resilience journey: "Learning to be resilient with MCAS meant accepting that some days would be harder than others and that wasn't my fault. I developed backup plans for everything - work, social activities, household tasks. Having options and support helped me feel more confident in my ability to handle whatever came up."

Recovery practices help you restore your energy and emotional balance after stressful periods. This might include rest, gentle movement, time in nature, creative activities, or spiritual practices. Regular recovery practices prevent stress from accumulating and overwhelming your coping capacity.

Growth mindset involves viewing challenges as opportunities for learning and development rather than threats to avoid. While you certainly didn't choose to have MCAS, you can choose to approach it as a teacher that's helping you develop skills, priorities, and perspectives that serve you well in all areas of life.

The Mind-Body Partnership

Managing MCAS effectively requires understanding that your mind and body are partners in both creating and resolving symptoms. The stress-mast cell connection isn't a weakness or character flaw - it's a biological reality that, once understood, provides powerful tools for symptom management and overall wellness.

The techniques and strategies you develop for stress management serve multiple purposes: they reduce stress-triggered symptoms, improve your quality of life, enhance your resilience for handling ongoing health challenges, and often provide benefits that extend far beyond MCAS management. Many people discover that the stress management skills they learn for MCAS improve their relationships, work performance, and overall life satisfaction.

Your nervous system has remarkable capacity for healing and adaptation when provided with consistent, gentle support. The same biological mechanisms that allow stress to trigger symptoms can be harnessed to promote calm, stability, and resilience. This partnership between conscious stress management efforts and unconscious nervous system responses creates powerful potential for both symptom relief and personal growth.

Key Learning Points

- Stress directly triggers mast cell activation through hormone release and nervous system pathways, making stress management essential for symptom control

- Nervous system dysregulation in MCAS affects autonomic functions and requires targeted support beyond typical stress management

- Stress reduction techniques including progressive muscle relaxation and deep breathing provide immediate and long-term benefits

- Mindfulness and meditation practices help you observe symptoms without adding the stress of resistance or fear

- Breathing techniques offer rapid, always-available tools for activating the parasympathetic nervous system

- Cognitive behavioral strategies help change thought patterns that increase stress and potentially trigger symptoms

- Building resilience creates lasting capacity for managing both daily stressors and MCAS-specific challenges

Chapter 10: Sleep Optimization for MCAS

- Restorative Sleep Despite Symptoms

The bedroom that once provided peaceful refuge now feels like another battleground where symptoms seem to intensify just when you need rest most. Your heart races as you try to settle into bed, your skin itches or burns without obvious cause, or digestive discomfort keeps you tossing and turning through the night. For many people with MCAS, sleep becomes both more necessary and more elusive, creating a frustrating cycle where poor sleep worsens symptoms, which then make sleep even more difficult to achieve.

Sleep represents one of the most critical components of MCAS management, yet it's often the most disrupted by the very condition it could help stabilize. Understanding why MCAS affects sleep and developing targeted strategies for improving sleep quality can dramatically impact your overall symptom control and quality of life. Quality sleep isn't a luxury when you have MCAS - it's medicine that supports mast cell stability, immune function, and nervous system regulation.

Sleep Disturbances in MCAS

MCAS can disrupt sleep through multiple mechanisms, creating a complex web of factors that interfere with both falling asleep and staying asleep. Understanding these mechanisms helps you develop targeted interventions that address the root causes rather than just treating the symptoms of poor sleep.

Histamine and sleep cycles interact in complex ways since histamine functions as both a wake-promoting neurotransmitter and an inflammatory mediator. Elevated histamine levels can directly interfere with sleep initiation and maintenance, while disrupted sleep can worsen histamine intolerance and mast cell stability. This creates a bidirectional relationship where sleep problems and MCAS symptoms reinforce each other (18).

Nighttime mast cell activation often occurs due to circadian changes in hormone levels, temperature fluctuations, or accumulated trigger exposure from the day. Many people experience their worst symptoms in the evening or during the night, when cortisol levels naturally drop and other regulatory mechanisms change. This timing can make bedtime particularly challenging.

Temperature regulation problems affect sleep quality since mast cell activation can disrupt normal thermoregulation. You might experience night sweats, feeling simultaneously hot and cold, or difficulty finding a comfortable temperature. Some people find they need to adjust their bedroom temperature throughout the night as their body's regulation systems fluctuate.

Cardiovascular symptoms including heart palpitations, rapid heart rate, or blood pressure fluctuations can make it difficult to relax enough for sleep. The sensation of your heart racing or beating irregularly can create anxiety that further interferes with sleep, even when the cardiovascular symptoms aren't dangerous.

Dr. Jennifer, a sleep medicine physician familiar with MCAS, explains: "Sleep problems in MCAS aren't just about histamine - they involve complex interactions between the immune system, nervous system, and circadian rhythms. Addressing sleep requires a multi-faceted approach that considers all these systems."

Respiratory symptoms can significantly impact sleep quality through nasal congestion, post-nasal drip, coughing, or a sensation of throat tightness. Some people experience sleep apnea or other breathing disruptions that may be related to inflammation in the upper airway tissues.

Pain and discomfort from various MCAS symptoms can make it difficult to find comfortable sleeping positions or stay asleep throughout the night. This might include joint pain, muscle aches, skin irritation, or gastrointestinal discomfort that worsens when lying down.

Anxiety and hypervigilance often develop around sleep, particularly after experiencing multiple nights of poor rest or nighttime reactions. The fear of not sleeping well can create enough anxiety to actually prevent good sleep, creating a self-fulfilling prophecy that's difficult to break.

Jennifer, a 35-year-old nurse, describes her sleep challenges: "My sleep problems started gradually - first just trouble falling asleep, then waking up multiple times during the night with my heart racing or feeling overheated. I began dreading bedtime because I never knew if I'd actually get rest or spend the night dealing with symptoms."

Sleep Hygiene Fundamentals

Establishing consistent sleep hygiene practices provides the foundation for better sleep quality, even when MCAS symptoms create additional challenges. These fundamental practices help optimize your sleep environment and routines to support natural sleep cycles while minimizing trigger exposures during rest periods.

Consistent sleep schedule helps regulate your circadian rhythms and can improve mast cell stability through better hormonal regulation. Try to go to bed and wake up at the same time every day, even on weekends. This consistency helps train your body's internal clock and can reduce the unpredictability that often characterizes MCAS symptoms.

Pre-sleep routines signal to your body that it's time to wind down and prepare for rest. Start your routine 1-2 hours before your intended bedtime, including activities that promote relaxation without triggering symptoms. This might include gentle stretching, reading, listening to calming music, or practicing relaxation techniques.

Screen time management becomes particularly important since blue light exposure can disrupt melatonin production and worsen sleep quality. Turn off electronic devices at least one hour before bedtime, or use blue light blocking glasses if you must use devices. Some people find that even small amounts of light from electronic devices can trigger sensitivity reactions.

Bedroom environment optimization involves creating a space that supports rest while minimizing potential triggers. Keep the room cool, dark, and quiet, but also ensure good air circulation and minimal chemical exposures from bedding, furniture, or air fresheners that might trigger nighttime reactions.

Caffeine and stimulant timing requires careful attention since people with MCAS may be more sensitive to stimulating substances or may metabolize them differently.

Avoid caffeine after 2 PM, and be aware that some people need to stop caffeine intake even earlier in the day to prevent sleep interference.

Mark, a 41-year-old engineer, improved his sleep through consistent routines: "I created a very structured bedtime routine and stuck to it religiously, even when I felt too wired to sleep. After about three weeks, my body started naturally getting tired around the same time each night, and my sleep quality improved significantly."

Exercise timing affects sleep quality, but the optimal timing varies between individuals with MCAS. Some people find that evening exercise helps them sleep better, while others discover that any activity within 3-4 hours of bedtime can trigger symptoms or make them too activated to rest.

Meal timing influences sleep quality since eating too close to bedtime can trigger digestive symptoms that interfere with rest. However, some people with MCAS find that having a small snack before bed helps stabilize their blood sugar and reduces nighttime symptoms.

Bedroom Environment Optimization

Creating an MCAS-friendly bedroom environment requires attention to factors that might not affect people without mast cell sensitivities. Your bedroom should serve as a sanctuary that supports rest while minimizing exposure to potential triggers that could disrupt sleep or cause nighttime reactions.

Air quality management starts with ensuring good ventilation while filtering out potential triggers. Use high-quality air purifiers with HEPA and carbon filtration to remove both particles and chemical vapors. Consider air purifiers specifically designed for bedrooms that operate quietly enough not to disturb sleep.

Temperature and humidity control help maintain optimal conditions for both sleep quality and mast cell stability. Most people sleep best in cooler temperatures (around 65-68°F), but individual preferences vary. Use humidity control to maintain levels between 40-50%, which reduces both mold growth and excessive dryness that might trigger respiratory symptoms.

Bedding selection should prioritize both comfort and trigger avoidance. Choose organic cotton, bamboo, or other natural fiber sheets that are less likely to contain chemical treatments or synthetic materials that might cause reactions. Wash new bedding multiple times before use to remove any residual chemicals.

Mattress considerations include both comfort and potential chemical exposures. Natural latex, organic cotton, or other low-chemical mattresses may be worth the investment if you're sensitive to the flame retardants, adhesives, or other chemicals used in conventional mattresses. Consider mattress covers that provide additional protection from dust mites and chemical exposures.

Lighting optimization involves minimizing light exposure during sleep while ensuring you can safely navigate your bedroom if needed during the night. Use blackout curtains or sleep masks to block external light, but consider small nightlights that won't disrupt sleep if you need to get up during the night.

Sarah, a 37-year-old teacher, transformed her bedroom environment: "I invested in an air purifier, organic cotton bedding, and blackout curtains. I also removed all fragranced products from my bedroom and started keeping my rescue medications and water on my nightstand. Having everything optimized for my MCAS needs made me feel safer and more relaxed at bedtime."

Sound management includes both minimizing disruptive noises and potentially adding beneficial sounds. Use earplugs, white noise machines, or fans to mask sudden sounds that might wake you. Some people find that consistent background sounds help them stay asleep even when symptoms cause mild discomfort.

Chemical exposure reduction extends beyond obvious sources like air fresheners to include cleaning products, laundry detergents, and personal care products used before bed. Use fragrance-free, chemical-free alternatives for anything that comes into contact with your bedroom environment.

Managing Nighttime Symptoms

Developing specific strategies for managing symptoms that occur during the night helps reduce their impact on sleep quality and prevents minor symptoms from escalating into major sleep disruptions. Having a plan for nighttime symptom management reduces anxiety and helps you respond effectively when symptoms occur.

Cardiovascular symptom management includes techniques for handling heart palpitations, rapid heart rate, or blood pressure fluctuations that occur during the night. Keep rescue medications easily accessible, practice calming breathing techniques, and consider elevating your head slightly if blood pressure drops cause dizziness when lying flat.

Temperature regulation strategies help manage hot flashes, night sweats, or feeling simultaneously hot and cold. Keep cooling packs in the freezer for quick relief, use moisture-wicking bedding materials, and consider layered bedding that you can easily adjust throughout the night.

Respiratory symptom relief might include keeping saline nasal sprays, humidifiers, or rescue inhalers accessible for nighttime congestion, coughing, or breathing difficulties. Elevating your head slightly can help with post-nasal drip or congestion that worsens when lying flat.

Gastrointestinal comfort measures for nighttime digestive symptoms might include keeping antacids or other safe remedies accessible, adjusting your sleeping position to minimize discomfort, or having small amounts of well-tolerated foods available if low blood sugar contributes to nighttime symptoms.

Skin irritation management for nighttime itching, burning, or other skin symptoms might include keeping cool, damp cloths available for relief, using gentle, fragrance-free moisturizers before bed, or wearing soft, natural fiber clothing that minimizes irritation.

Lisa, a 33-year-old marketing manager, developed effective nighttime protocols: "I keep a 'symptom kit' on my nightstand with everything I might need - extra antihistamines, cooling packs, saline spray, antacids, and a small water bottle. Having everything within reach means I don't have to fully wake up or get out of bed when symptoms occur, which helps me get back to sleep faster."

Positioning strategies can help minimize symptom severity and improve comfort during sleep. Some people find that sleeping slightly elevated helps with cardiovascular symptoms or respiratory issues. Side sleeping might reduce gastrointestinal symptoms for some people, while others need to experiment with different positions based on their symptom patterns.

Calm response protocols help prevent nighttime symptoms from triggering anxiety that makes sleep more difficult. Practice relaxation techniques that you can use when symptoms occur, focus on staying calm rather than fighting the symptoms, and remind yourself that nighttime symptoms often resolve on their own or with gentle interventions.

Sleep Medications and MCAS

Medication approaches to sleep problems in MCAS require careful consideration of both effectiveness and potential sensitivity reactions. Many conventional sleep medications can interact with MCAS treatments or may not be well-tolerated by people with sensitive immune systems.

Antihistamine sleep aids like diphenhydramine (Benadryl) or doxylamine can provide dual benefits by promoting sleep while also blocking histamine receptors. However, these medications can cause next-day grogginess, and some people develop tolerance over time. They may be most useful for occasional use rather than nightly sleep support.

Prescription sleep medications including zolpidem (Ambien), eszopiclone (Lunesta), or other sleep aids may be necessary for some people with severe sleep disruption. Work with your healthcare provider to identify medications that are least likely to interact with your MCAS treatments or trigger sensitivity reactions.

Natural sleep aids might include melatonin, magnesium, valerian root, or other supplements that support sleep. However, people with MCAS may be sensitive to certain supplements or may need to start with very small doses to assess tolerance. Some herbal sleep aids can interact with medications or trigger reactions in sensitive individuals.

Timing considerations for sleep medications become important when you're taking multiple medications for MCAS management. Some sleep aids should not be taken with certain antihistamines or other MCAS medications. Work with your pharmacist and healthcare provider to optimize timing and avoid interactions.

Dr. Michael, a psychiatrist familiar with MCAS, notes: "Sleep medication selection for MCAS patients requires balancing effectiveness with sensitivity concerns. We often start with very low doses and increase gradually while monitoring for both sleep improvement and any adverse reactions."

Medication-free approaches may be preferable for some people who are highly sensitive to medications or who prefer to minimize pharmaceutical interventions. These might include cognitive behavioral therapy for insomnia, relaxation training, or other behavioral interventions that can improve sleep quality without medication.

Withdrawal considerations become important if you've been using sleep medications long-term and want to reduce or discontinue them. Work with your healthcare provider to develop a gradual tapering plan that prevents rebound insomnia while maintaining your MCAS symptom control.

Circadian Rhythm Support

Supporting healthy circadian rhythms can significantly improve sleep quality while also stabilizing many MCAS symptoms that fluctuate with daily hormone and neurotransmitter cycles. Your internal clock influences immune function, stress hormone production, and mast cell stability throughout the day.

Light exposure timing helps regulate your circadian clock through its effects on melatonin production and other hormones. Get bright light exposure in the morning, preferably from natural sunlight, and minimize bright light exposure in the evening. This helps maintain the natural rhythm of alertness during the day and sleepiness at night.

Meal timing influences circadian rhythms through metabolic pathways that communicate with your central clock. Try to eat your largest meals earlier in the day and avoid large meals close to bedtime. Some people benefit from small, well-tolerated snacks in the evening to prevent blood sugar drops that can disrupt sleep.

Activity scheduling should align with your natural energy patterns when possible. Many people with MCAS find they have optimal energy windows during certain parts of the day. Schedule demanding activities during these peak periods and plan for rest during naturally low-energy times.

Hormone support might involve melatonin supplementation, though the timing and dosing require careful consideration. Some people benefit from very small doses of melatonin taken 2-3 hours before bedtime, while others find that melatonin disrupts their sleep or causes next-day grogginess.

Jennifer, a 39-year-old accountant, improved her circadian rhythms: "I started getting morning sunlight exposure by having my coffee outside for 15 minutes each day and avoiding screens after 9 PM. I also shifted my largest meal to lunchtime instead of dinner. These changes helped regulate my sleep-wake cycle and reduced my nighttime MCAS symptoms."

Consistency maintenance becomes particularly important during times of stress, illness, or schedule disruption when circadian rhythms are more vulnerable to disruption. Try to maintain regular sleep and wake times even during challenging periods, as consistent rhythms can help stabilize other MCAS symptoms.

Seasonal adjustments may be necessary as daylight patterns change throughout the year. Some people with MCAS find their symptoms and sleep patterns shift with seasonal changes. Light therapy, vitamin D supplementation, or other seasonal support strategies might be helpful during darker months.

Sleep Tracking and Assessment

Monitoring your sleep patterns and quality helps identify factors that improve or worsen your rest while providing objective information about the relationship between sleep and your MCAS symptoms. Effective tracking doesn't require expensive technology - simple observation and record-keeping can provide valuable information.

Sleep diary maintenance involves tracking bedtime, wake time, time to fall asleep, number of nighttime awakenings, overall sleep quality, and any symptoms that occurred during the night. Also note factors that might influence sleep such as stress levels, trigger exposures, medication timing, or environmental conditions.

Symptom correlation tracking helps identify patterns between sleep quality and MCAS symptom severity. Many people discover that poor sleep reliably leads to increased symptoms the following day, while good sleep provides protection against triggers and improves overall stability.

Environmental factor documentation includes room temperature, humidity levels, air quality, noise levels, and any potential trigger exposures in the bedroom. This information helps you optimize your sleep environment and identify factors that consistently improve or worsen your rest.

Medication and supplement effects should be tracked to identify which interventions help your sleep and which might cause problems. Note the timing, dosage, and effects of any sleep aids, MCAS medications, or supplements that might influence your rest.

Michael, a 43-year-old teacher, found tracking revelatory: "I kept a sleep diary for three months and discovered that my worst sleep always followed high-stress days or exposure to certain environmental triggers. I also realized that taking my evening antihistamine earlier improved my sleep quality. The tracking helped me identify patterns I never would have noticed otherwise."

Technology considerations for sleep tracking include wearable devices, smartphone apps, or other tools that can provide objective sleep data. However, some people with

MCAS are sensitive to electromagnetic fields or find that wearing devices disrupts their sleep. Choose tracking methods that don't add stress or trigger symptoms.

Pattern identification involves looking for trends in your sleep data over time rather than focusing on individual nights. Look for factors that consistently improve sleep, trigger patterns that disrupt rest, and overall trends in sleep quality as your MCAS management improves.

Rest as Foundation

Quality sleep forms the foundation upon which all other MCAS management strategies build. When you're well-rested, your immune system functions more effectively, your stress tolerance improves, and your overall resilience against triggers increases. Conversely, poor sleep can undermine even the best dietary, medication, and stress management efforts.

The investment you make in optimizing your sleep pays dividends that extend far beyond feeling more rested. Better sleep can reduce medication needs, improve your ability to handle dietary flexibility, increase your tolerance for environmental exposures, and significantly enhance your quality of life. Many people find that addressing sleep problems provides more symptom relief than any other single intervention.

Your sleep needs and optimal strategies may change over time as your MCAS management improves or as life circumstances shift. The skills you develop in creating supportive sleep environments and managing nighttime symptoms will serve you well throughout these changes, providing a stable foundation for ongoing health and wellness.

Key Insights for Better Rest

- MCAS disrupts sleep through histamine elevation, temperature dysregulation, and cardiovascular symptoms that interfere with natural sleep cycles

- Sleep hygiene fundamentals including consistent schedules and pre-sleep routines provide essential foundation for better rest

- Bedroom environment optimization requires attention to air quality, temperature control, and chemical exposure reduction

- Nighttime symptom management strategies help minimize sleep disruption when MCAS symptoms occur during rest periods

- Sleep medications for MCAS require careful selection and timing to avoid interactions and sensitivity reactions

- Circadian rhythm support through light exposure and meal timing can stabilize both sleep patterns and MCAS symptoms

- Sleep tracking and assessment help identify effective interventions and patterns between rest quality and symptom control

Chapter 11: Travel and Social Navigation

- Maintaining Your Life Activities

The wedding invitation arrives with its beautiful calligraphy and promises of celebration, but your first thought isn't about what to wear or how much fun you'll have. Instead, you find yourself calculating the risks: Will there be strong fragrances from flowers or perfumes? Can you eat safely at the reception? What if you have a reaction away from home? For people with MCAS, social events and travel require careful planning that goes far beyond what most people consider, yet maintaining these connections and experiences remains essential for your overall well-being and quality of life.

Living with MCAS doesn't mean retreating from the world or missing out on meaningful experiences. It means developing new skills for planning, communicating, and adapting so you can participate safely in the activities that matter most to you. With thoughtful preparation and clear communication strategies, you can maintain relationships, travel to new places, and engage in social activities while managing your health needs effectively.

Travel Planning and Preparation

Successful travel with MCAS requires systematic planning that addresses potential triggers, ensures access to safe foods and medications, and prepares for emergency situations in unfamiliar locations. The key is thinking through every aspect of your trip before you leave home, creating backup plans for common problems, and carrying everything you need to manage your condition away from your usual support systems.

Destination research starts months before your departure date. Investigate the climate conditions you'll encounter, including temperature ranges, humidity levels, and seasonal allergen patterns. Research local air quality conditions and pollution levels, particularly if you're sensitive to environmental triggers. Look into local healthcare facilities and emergency services in case you need medical attention during your trip.

Accommodation selection requires more than just reading standard hotel reviews. Contact hotels directly to ask about their cleaning products, air freshener policies, and room preparation procedures. Request rooms that haven't been recently painted, carpeted, or treated with pest control chemicals. Some hotel chains offer allergy-friendly rooms with improved air filtration and chemical-free cleaning protocols.

Ask for rooms away from smoking areas, pools with heavy chlorine use, or high-traffic areas where you might encounter more fragrances and chemical exposures. Request that housekeeping avoid using air fresheners, fabric sprays, or other scented products in your room during your stay.

Medication management becomes particularly critical when traveling since you won't have easy access to pharmacies or healthcare providers familiar with your condition. Bring more medications than you think you'll need - pack at least a week's extra supply of all essential medications. Carry medications in their original bottles with pharmacy labels to avoid problems with security screening.

Keep emergency medications in your carry-on bag and easily accessible during travel. This includes rescue inhalers, epinephrine auto-injectors, extra antihistamines, and any other medications you might need for acute reactions. Consider carrying a letter from your doctor explaining your condition and medication needs in case you encounter questions from security personnel.

Sarah, a 39-year-old nurse, learned to travel systematically: "I created a detailed travel checklist that covers everything from researching the destination's air quality to packing extra medications and safe food options. I also scout out the nearest hospital and urgent care facilities before I even book my trip. The planning takes time, but it gives me confidence to travel knowing I'm prepared for different scenarios."

Food planning requires researching safe dining options at your destination and bringing backup foods for emergencies. Contact restaurants in advance to discuss your dietary restrictions and ask about ingredient lists and preparation methods. Research grocery stores near your accommodation where you can buy safe foods and snacks.

Pack non-perishable safe foods that can sustain you if local options aren't suitable. This might include safe snacks, meal replacement options, or specialty products that you can't find at your destination. Consider bringing a small cooler for perishable items if you're traveling by car.

Emergency contact information should include your healthcare providers at home, local emergency services at your destination, and any contacts who can help coordinate care if needed. Carry this information in multiple formats - written copies, in your phone, and with your travel companions.

Transportation Considerations

Different modes of transportation present unique challenges and opportunities for people with MCAS. Understanding these differences helps you choose the best options for your specific triggers and prepare effectively for the journey itself, not just the destination.

Air travel requires the most extensive preparation due to limited control over the cabin environment and difficulty accessing help during flights. Research airline policies regarding medical equipment, medication storage, and food restrictions. Some airlines allow you to pre-board to wipe down your seating area and minimize exposure to cleaning chemicals used between flights.

Request seat assignments away from bathrooms, where air fresheners are commonly used, and galleys, where food preparation might trigger reactions. Consider aisle seats for easier access to bathrooms and the ability to stand and move if needed. Window seats provide some isolation from other passengers but make it harder to leave your seat quickly.

Pack a travel air purifier designed for personal use if you're sensitive to airborne triggers. Bring masks that filter both particles and some chemical vapors. Consider noise-canceling headphones to reduce sensory overwhelm that might contribute to stress-triggered reactions.

Car travel offers the most control over your environment but requires careful planning for longer trips. Ensure your vehicle's air filtration system is working properly and consider upgrading to higher-quality cabin air filters. Plan routes that avoid high-pollution areas when possible, and identify safe stopping points for meals and rest breaks.

Pack a cooler with safe foods and drinks for the journey, and research restaurants along your route that can accommodate your dietary needs. Bring cleaning supplies to wipe down hotel surfaces if you're staying overnight during a road trip.

Train and bus travel fall somewhere between air and car travel in terms of environmental control. These modes often have better air circulation than cars but less control than flying. Research policies about food, medications, and any accommodations available for passengers with medical needs.

Michael, a 42-year-old teacher, mastered car travel strategies: "I plan my driving routes to avoid major cities during rush hour when air pollution is worst, and I research safe restaurant stops along the way. I keep my emergency kit easily accessible in the car and always travel with a cooler of safe foods and drinks. Having control over my environment makes car travel my preferred option for longer trips."

Public transportation in urban areas requires strategies for managing crowd exposures, air quality, and limited control over environmental conditions. Plan travel during off-peak hours when possible to reduce crowding and exposure to multiple fragrances and chemicals. Carry portable air purifiers or masks designed for public transportation use.

Accommodation Safety

Creating a safe environment in hotels, vacation rentals, or other temporary accommodations requires immediate assessment and modification of your surroundings. Unlike your carefully controlled home environment, temporary accommodations may expose you to numerous triggers that require quick identification and mitigation.

Room assessment should begin immediately upon arrival. Check for obvious sources of strong scents like air fresheners, scented cleaning products, or recent carpet cleaning. Open windows if possible to air out the room and reduce chemical concentrations. Look for signs of mold, water damage, or pest control treatments that might trigger reactions.

Test the air conditioning and heating systems to ensure they're working properly and not circulating stale or chemically-treated air. Some people need to run the ventilation system for several hours with windows open to clear out accumulated chemicals before the room becomes tolerable.

Room modification strategies help create a safer immediate environment. Remove or unplug air fresheners, scented products, and any items that trigger your sensitivities. Wipe down surfaces with your own safe cleaning products to remove residual chemicals from hotel cleaning supplies.

Set up your portable air purifier immediately and position it near your sleeping area for maximum benefit. If you brought your own bedding or pillowcases, replace the hotel linens with your familiar, safe materials.

Communication with staff can help prevent problems and address issues that arise during your stay. Inform housekeeping about your chemical sensitivities and request that they avoid using air fresheners, fabric sprays, or heavily scented cleaning products in your room. Ask that they use minimal cleaning products and ensure good ventilation during room cleaning.

Request that pest control treatments, carpet cleaning, or painting not be scheduled near your room during your stay. Many hotels are willing to accommodate these requests when they understand the medical necessity.

Jennifer, a 35-year-old marketing manager, developed effective accommodation strategies: "I always travel with a small bottle of safe all-purpose cleaner and immediately wipe down surfaces in my hotel room. I set up my air purifier right away and open windows to air out the space. I also call the front desk to request no housekeeping services unless I specifically ask for them, which prevents unexpected chemical exposures."

Backup accommodation plans prepare you for situations where your primary accommodation becomes unsuitable due to unexpected chemical exposures, nearby construction, or other unforeseen circumstances. Research alternative hotels or vacation rentals in the area and keep contact information readily available.

Consider travel insurance that covers accommodation changes due to medical needs, though this coverage varies significantly between policies and may require documentation of your condition.

Social Event Navigation

Attending social events with MCAS requires balancing your health needs with your desire to participate in meaningful social experiences. Successful navigation involves advance planning, clear communication with hosts, and flexible strategies that allow you to participate safely while maintaining important relationships.

Event planning conversations with hosts help set realistic expectations and identify potential accommodations. Contact hosts well in advance to discuss your dietary restrictions, sensitivity to fragrances, and any other needs that might affect your participation. Most hosts are happy to make reasonable accommodations when they understand the medical nature of your requests.

Ask about the menu and whether ingredients lists are available for dishes being served. Inquire about the venue's ventilation, whether flowers or strongly scented decorations will be used, and if guests typically wear fragrances to such events.

Strategic participation allows you to attend events while minimizing exposure to triggers. Plan to arrive after initial setup activities that might involve cleaning products or floral arrangements. Consider leaving before cleanup activities that might involve strong chemicals or increased dust and allergen disturbance.

Position yourself near exits or areas with good ventilation where you can easily leave if needed. Avoid crowded areas where you might be exposed to multiple fragrances or have difficulty leaving quickly if symptoms develop.

Safe eating strategies help you enjoy food-centered social events while avoiding dietary triggers. Offer to bring a dish you can safely eat, ensuring you'll have at least one safe option available. Eat a small safe meal before attending events where food options might be limited.

Ask hosts about ingredients and preparation methods for dishes you're considering. When in doubt, politely decline foods that might contain triggers rather than risking a reaction during the event.

Mark, a 44-year-old engineer, found success with social events: "I learned to be upfront with hosts about my needs, and most people are very accommodating. I always bring a dish I can eat and position myself near windows or doors for fresh air access. I also set a specific time limit for how long I'll stay, which helps me leave before I get overwhelmed rather than pushing through and risking a reaction."

Gift and celebration considerations extend your social navigation skills to gift-giving occasions and celebrations. Choose fragrance-free gifts and cards for others, and communicate your own sensitivities to friends and family who might give you scented products.

For celebrations in your honor, provide hosts with specific suggestions for safe decorations, foods, and venue considerations that allow you to fully enjoy events celebrating milestones in your life.

Communicating About MCAS

Effective communication about your condition helps others understand your needs while maintaining relationships and reducing the stress of constantly explaining or defending your health requirements. Developing clear, concise explanations for different audiences and situations makes social interactions smoother and more successful.

Elevator explanations provide brief, clear descriptions of your condition for casual social situations. Develop 30-second explanations that cover the essential points without overwhelming listeners with medical details. Focus on practical implications rather than complex pathophysiology.

For example: "I have a condition called MCAS where my immune system overreacts to everyday things like fragrances and certain foods. I need to be careful about what I eat and avoid strong scents, but with some planning, I can participate in most activities."

Detailed explanations work better for close friends, family members, or employers who need to understand your condition more thoroughly. These conversations allow you to explain the unpredictable nature of symptoms, the importance of avoiding triggers, and specific ways others can help support your participation in shared activities.

Include information about how stress and environmental factors can affect your symptoms, why certain accommodations are necessary, and what emergency situations might look like so others can recognize when you need help.

Written communication can be helpful for formal situations like workplace accommodations, school settings, or medical situations where precise information is important. Having written explanations available saves you from repeatedly explaining your condition and ensures consistent, accurate information is shared.

Boundary setting becomes necessary when people don't understand or respect your health needs. Practice polite but firm responses for common challenging situations, such as people who insist their fragrance isn't strong or pressure you to eat foods you know will trigger reactions.

Sarah, a 38-year-old accountant, developed effective communication strategies: "I found that most people respond well when I give them concrete ways to help rather than just explaining what I can't do. Instead of saying 'I can't be around fragrances,' I say 'I'd love to come to your party - would it be possible to ask guests to go easy on perfumes and cologne?' Most people are happy to help when they know how."

Advocacy without exhaustion involves choosing your battles wisely and conserving emotional energy for situations where education and advocacy are most likely to be effective. You don't need to educate every person you encounter about MCAS, and sometimes brief explanations or polite deflection work better than detailed medical discussions.

Maintaining Relationships

Living with MCAS can strain relationships as your needs change and social participation becomes more complex. Maintaining strong connections requires honest communication, mutual understanding, and often some relationship adaptation as you learn to balance health needs with social desires.

Friendship evolution often occurs as you learn to manage MCAS and discover which friends are supportive of your health needs versus those who minimize or dismiss your condition. Quality becomes more important than quantity as you invest energy in relationships with people who respect your boundaries and support your well-being.

Some friendships may naturally fade as activities become more challenging or as friends become frustrated with accommodation needs. This process, while sometimes painful, often leads to stronger, more authentic relationships with people who truly understand and support you.

Family dynamics require particular attention since family relationships are often long-term and emotionally significant. Family members may need time to understand your condition and adjust their expectations for family gatherings, holiday traditions, and shared activities.

Some family members may be more supportive than others, and you might need to set different boundaries with different relatives based on their understanding and willingness to accommodate your needs. Focus your energy on relationships that are reciprocal and supportive rather than trying to convince skeptical family members of the validity of your condition.

Romantic relationships face unique challenges when MCAS affects daily life, social activities, and future planning. Open communication about your health needs, the unpredictable nature of symptoms, and the importance of having a supportive partner becomes essential for relationship success.

Partners need to understand that your condition is real, that symptoms aren't choices or character flaws, and that accommodation needs are medical necessities rather than preferences. The best partnerships involve mutual problem-solving and flexibility in adapting shared activities to support both partners' needs.

Lisa, a 36-year-old teacher, learned to prioritize supportive relationships: "I realized I was spending too much energy trying to maintain friendships with people who didn't really understand or support my health needs. When I started focusing on the friends who were willing to meet at fragrance-free venues or host gatherings with my dietary needs in mind, my social life actually improved even though I saw fewer people overall."

Creating new connections often becomes necessary as your social needs and capabilities change with MCAS management. Look for communities and activities that naturally align with your health needs, such as outdoor activities in clean air environments, cooking classes focused on whole foods, or support groups for people with chronic health conditions.

Online communities can provide valuable social connections that don't require physical presence and exposure to environmental triggers. Many people find meaningful friendships through MCAS support groups, health-focused forums, or shared interest groups that accommodate various health needs.

Workplace Accommodations

Professional environments present unique challenges for MCAS management since you have limited control over air quality, chemical exposures, and food options while needing to maintain job performance and professional relationships. Understanding your rights and developing effective accommodation strategies helps you succeed professionally while protecting your health.

Legal protections under the Americans with Disabilities Act (ADA) and similar laws may apply to workplace accommodations for MCAS, though the extent of coverage depends on how significantly your condition affects major life activities and your ability to perform job functions. Documentation from healthcare providers can support accommodation requests.

Common accommodations for MCAS in workplace settings include fragrance-free policies for your immediate work area, permission to use air purifiers at your desk, flexible scheduling for medical appointments, and the ability to work from home during high symptom periods or when building maintenance activities might trigger reactions.

Other accommodations might include parking closer to entrances to minimize exposure during commutes, access to refrigeration for medications that require cooling, or modified break schedules to allow for medication timing around meals.

Communication strategies with supervisors and human resources focus on specific job performance needs rather than detailed medical explanations. Emphasize how accommodations will help you maintain productivity and attendance rather than focusing primarily on symptom management.

Provide concrete examples of accommodations that would be helpful and explain how they relate to your ability to perform your job effectively. Many employers are more receptive to accommodation requests when they understand the connection to job performance and see that you're taking initiative to solve potential problems.

Michael, a 41-year-old project manager, successfully obtained workplace accommodations: "I approached my supervisor with specific solutions rather than just problems. I explained that an air purifier at my desk and a fragrance-free policy in our department would help me maintain consistent attendance and productivity. When they saw I had practical solutions that didn't burden the company, they were very supportive."

Documentation requirements for workplace accommodations typically include letters from healthcare providers describing your condition, its impact on major life activities, and specific recommendations for workplace modifications. Work with your healthcare team to provide clear, professional documentation that supports your requests.

Remote work considerations have become more common and can provide excellent accommodations for people with MCAS who can perform their job duties from home. Remote work eliminates many environmental triggers while allowing you to control your workspace completely.

Emergency Planning Away from Home

Preparing for medical emergencies while traveling or attending social events requires additional planning beyond your usual emergency protocols. Being away from familiar healthcare providers and emergency services means you need to be more self-sufficient while having clear plans for accessing help when needed.

Emergency kit adaptation for travel should include everything in your home emergency kit plus additional supplies for extended periods away from home. Pack extra rescue medications, emergency contact information for healthcare providers at home and at your destination, and copies of important medical records.

Include a thermometer, blood pressure monitor if you use one, and any medical devices you might need for monitoring symptoms or delivering treatments. Pack these items in easily accessible locations and carry essential items with you rather than packing everything in checked luggage.

Local emergency preparation involves researching emergency services at your destination before you travel. Identify the nearest hospital emergency departments, urgent care centers, and pharmacies. Save important phone numbers in your cell phone and carry written copies as backup.

Research which hospitals have emergency departments experienced with allergic reactions and anaphylaxis treatment. Some areas have limited medical facilities, making this research particularly important for travel to rural or remote locations.

Communication planning ensures that people at home know your travel plans and can help coordinate care if needed. Provide detailed itineraries to trusted family members or friends, including accommodation information, planned activities, and local emergency contact numbers.

Consider medical alert services that can coordinate emergency care when you're traveling, particularly for international travel where language barriers might complicate emergency situations.

Jennifer, a 33-year-old nurse, developed comprehensive emergency travel planning: "I create a travel emergency packet for every trip that includes copies of my medical records, current medication lists, emergency contact information, and details about local medical facilities. I share this information with my family and keep copies in multiple locations during travel. It gives me confidence to travel knowing I'm prepared for medical emergencies."

Insurance coordination becomes particularly important for travel, especially international travel where your regular insurance coverage might not apply. Research your insurance coverage for emergency care away from home and consider supplemental travel insurance that covers medical emergencies and evacuation if needed.

Understand what documentation your insurance requires for emergency care and carry necessary insurance cards and contact information with you during travel.

The Art of Adaptive Living

Living fully with MCAS requires developing skills that most people never need to learn - the art of participating in life while carefully managing health needs that others can't see or understand. This adaptation isn't about limitation; it's about developing sophisticated strategies that allow you to maintain the relationships and experiences that give your life meaning while protecting the health that makes those experiences possible.

The planning and communication skills you develop for managing social situations and travel with MCAS often improve your life in unexpected ways. Many people discover they become more intentional about their social choices, more appreciative of supportive relationships, and more skilled at problem-solving and advance planning in all areas of life.

Your experience managing MCAS in social and travel situations also positions you to help others facing similar challenges. The strategies you develop and the grace you learn to show yourself in adapting to health needs can inspire and guide others who are learning to live fully with chronic health conditions.

Essential Strategies for Social Success

- Travel planning requires researching destinations, preparing accommodations, and packing comprehensive medication and emergency supplies

- Transportation choices should consider environmental control, air quality, and access to emergency assistance during transit

- Accommodation safety involves immediate assessment and modification of temporary living spaces to reduce trigger exposures

- Social event navigation balances participation desires with health needs through advance planning and strategic positioning

- Communication about MCAS requires developing clear explanations tailored to different audiences and relationship contexts

- Maintaining relationships focuses on quality over quantity while building connections with people who support your health needs

- Workplace accommodations involve understanding legal protections and requesting specific modifications that support job performance

- Emergency planning away from home requires comprehensive preparation for medical situations in unfamiliar locations

Chapter 12: Emergency Planning and Crisis Management

- Preparing for and Managing Severe Reactions

The moment you realize a mild reaction is escalating into something more serious changes everything. Your carefully managed daily routine suddenly feels inadequate as symptoms intensify beyond your usual coping strategies. Your heart pounds not just from the reaction itself, but from the fear of not knowing how severe this episode might become or if you're prepared to handle it effectively. For people with MCAS, developing robust emergency planning isn't just prudent preparation - it's an essential life skill that can mean the difference between a manageable crisis and a life-threatening situation.

Emergency preparedness for MCAS extends beyond knowing when to call 911. It involves recognizing the early warning signs of escalating reactions, having immediate access to appropriate treatments, and maintaining clear communication systems that ensure you receive proper care even when you can't advocate for yourself. The goal isn't to live in fear of severe reactions, but to build confidence through thorough preparation that allows you to respond effectively when serious situations arise.

Recognizing Medical Emergencies

Understanding the difference between manageable MCAS symptoms and true medical emergencies requires developing awareness of escalation patterns and recognizing when home management strategies aren't sufficient. This recognition often involves subtle changes in symptom quality or intensity rather than obvious dramatic presentations.

Cardiovascular emergency signs include heart rates that remain extremely elevated (over 130 beats per minute) despite rest and calming techniques, chest pain that feels different from your typical MCAS chest discomfort, blood pressure drops that cause sustained dizziness or fainting, or any combination of cardiovascular symptoms that doesn't respond to your usual interventions within 15-20 minutes.

Pay attention to changes in your heart rhythm, particularly irregular beating patterns or the sensation that your heart is skipping beats frequently. While occasional palpitations are common in MCAS, persistent irregular rhythms warrant immediate medical evaluation.

Respiratory emergency indicators include difficulty breathing that worsens progressively, wheezing that doesn't improve with rescue inhalers, the sensation of throat closure or swelling, voice changes that suggest airway involvement, or any breathing difficulty that interferes with speaking in complete sentences.

Systemic emergency patterns often involve multiple body systems showing severe symptoms simultaneously. This might include cardiovascular symptoms combined with severe gastrointestinal distress and neurological changes, or skin reactions that spread rapidly while breathing difficulties develop.

Neurological warning signs include confusion, severe dizziness that doesn't improve with sitting or lying down, vision changes, severe headaches that feel different from your typical MCAS headaches, or any level of consciousness change that makes it difficult to think clearly or communicate effectively.

Dr. Rachel, an emergency medicine physician experienced with MCAS, explains: "The key to recognizing MCAS emergencies is understanding your personal baseline and recognizing when symptoms exceed your usual patterns. A heart rate of 120 might be normal for one patient's reactions but could indicate a serious emergency for another patient who typically stays below 100."

Progressive worsening patterns often provide more reliable emergency indicators than absolute symptom levels. If symptoms continue worsening despite appropriate interventions, or if new symptoms keep appearing every few minutes, these patterns suggest the need for emergency care even if individual symptoms don't seem severe.

Failure to respond to usual treatments can indicate that a reaction has progressed beyond home management capabilities. If your typical rescue medications aren't providing relief within their usual timeframe, or if symptoms return quickly after initial improvement, emergency evaluation may be necessary.

Sarah, a 37-year-old teacher, learned to recognize her emergency patterns: "I used to wait too long to seek help because my emergency symptoms weren't like the textbook descriptions of anaphylaxis. I learned to trust my instinct when symptoms felt different or weren't responding to my usual treatments. Now I go to the ER when my gut tells me something is seriously wrong, even if I can't put my finger on exactly what's different."

Documentation during emergencies helps both your immediate care and future emergency planning. If possible, note the time symptoms started, what you were exposed to before symptoms began, which treatments you've tried and their effects, and the progression of symptoms over time. This information helps emergency providers understand your situation more quickly.

Anaphylaxis Recognition and Treatment

Anaphylaxis represents the most severe form of mast cell activation and requires immediate recognition and treatment. For people with MCAS, anaphylaxis may present differently than classic textbook descriptions, making personal awareness of your individual patterns particularly important.

Anaphylaxis criteria for people with MCAS may be met when severe symptoms affect two or more body systems simultaneously, when cardiovascular collapse occurs regardless of other symptoms, or when respiratory symptoms threaten breathing adequacy. The progression can be rapid or gradual, and symptoms may not follow typical patterns.

Skin involvement in anaphylaxis often includes widespread hives, severe itching, flushing that covers large areas of the body, or swelling of the face, lips, tongue, or throat. However, some people experience anaphylaxis without significant skin symptoms, particularly if cardiovascular or respiratory systems are primarily affected.

Cardiovascular anaphylaxis may present as severe drops in blood pressure, fainting or near-fainting episodes, rapid weak pulse, or cardiovascular symptoms that develop quickly and don't respond to position changes or usual interventions. Some people experience cardiovascular collapse as their primary anaphylaxis presentation.

Respiratory anaphylaxis includes severe shortness of breath, wheezing, voice changes, sensation of throat closure, or difficulty swallowing. Respiratory symptoms in anaphylaxis often progress rapidly and may not respond well to typical asthma treatments.

Gastrointestinal anaphylaxis can include severe nausea and vomiting, intense abdominal cramping, diarrhea, or a combination of digestive symptoms that occur suddenly and severely. While GI symptoms alone rarely constitute anaphylaxis, they often accompany other system involvement.

Michael, a 43-year-old engineer, experienced his first anaphylaxis episode: "I thought I was just having a bad MCAS day until my blood pressure dropped and I nearly fainted. The combination of my usual symptoms plus the cardiovascular collapse made me realize this was different from my typical reactions. Having epinephrine available and knowing how to use it probably saved my life."

Epinephrine administration represents the first-line treatment for anaphylaxis and should be given immediately when anaphylaxis is suspected. Don't delay epinephrine while waiting to see if symptoms improve - early administration is safer and more effective than delayed treatment.

Epinephrine auto-injectors should be carried by anyone with MCAS who has experienced severe reactions or who has risk factors for anaphylaxis. Learn proper injection technique and practice with trainer devices so you can administer the medication quickly during an emergency.

Post-epinephrine care requires immediate emergency medical attention even if symptoms improve after epinephrine administration. Epinephrine effects are temporary, and biphasic reactions can occur hours after initial improvement. Call 911 immediately after giving epinephrine and go to the emergency department for monitoring and additional treatment.

Emergency Action Plans

Written emergency action plans provide clear guidance for you and others during medical crises when clear thinking may be impaired by symptoms, stress, or treatments. These plans should be easily accessible and regularly updated to reflect changes in your condition or treatment approach.

Personal emergency protocols should include step-by-step instructions for recognizing emergencies, administering rescue medications, and accessing emergency care. Write these instructions in clear, simple language that you or others can follow during stressful situations.

Include specific criteria for when to take each rescue medication, when to call emergency services, and when to contact your healthcare providers. Make the decision-making process as clear as possible to avoid confusion during emergencies.

Medication administration schedules should specify which medications to take in what order and timing during escalating reactions. Some people benefit from graduated response plans that outline mild, moderate, and severe reaction protocols with specific interventions for each level.

Include dosing information for all rescue medications, timing between doses, and maximum safe doses in a given time period. Specify when to repeat doses and when medication failure indicates the need for emergency services.

Emergency contact hierarchies should list who to call in different emergency scenarios. This might include your emergency contact person, your primary healthcare provider, specialists familiar with your condition, and emergency services. Include both phone numbers and relationship information so emergency responders understand who they're contacting.

Jennifer, a 35-year-old marketing manager, developed a comprehensive action plan: "My emergency plan has three levels - yellow for moderate reactions, orange for severe reactions, and red for anaphylaxis. Each level has specific medications, timing, and decision points for when to escalate care. I keep copies in my purse, car, at home, and at work so it's always accessible."

Communication templates help others advocate for you when you can't communicate effectively yourself. These might include brief medical summaries, current medication lists, and specific information about your condition that emergency providers should know.

Include information about medications that have caused problems, effective treatments from previous emergencies, and any special considerations for your care. Keep this information current and easily accessible to emergency contacts.

Location-specific plans account for different emergency scenarios at home, work, while traveling, or in other common locations. Each setting may require different approaches based on available resources, proximity to medical care, and support people who might be present.

Emergency Kit Essentials

Emergency kits for MCAS must be portable enough to carry regularly while containing everything needed to manage severe reactions until professional help arrives. The contents should be organized for quick access during stressful situations and regularly checked for expiration dates and functionality.

Medication essentials include epinephrine auto-injectors (carry at least two), rescue inhalers if you have respiratory symptoms, extra antihistamines in fast-acting forms, anti-nausea medications, and any other rescue medications prescribed specifically for emergencies.

Store medications in temperature-controlled environments and replace them before expiration dates. Consider carrying both auto-injectors and traditional epinephrine if your healthcare provider recommends this approach for severe reactions.

Medical information should include current medication lists, emergency contact information, brief medical history, insurance information, and copies of important medical records. Store this information in waterproof containers and keep it updated regularly.

Include medical alert information, healthcare provider contact details, and any specific instructions for your emergency care. Consider medical alert jewelry or cards that provide basic information even if you can't communicate.

Monitoring equipment might include a thermometer, blood pressure monitor if you use one regularly, pulse oximeter if recommended by your healthcare provider, and any other devices that help assess your condition during reactions.

Communication tools ensure you can contact help even when traveling or in areas with poor cell service. This might include charged cell phones, emergency contact cards, medical alert devices, or satellite communication devices for remote travel.

Mark, a 44-year-old accountant, optimized his emergency kit: "I keep emergency kits in my car, at work, and carry one with me everywhere. Each kit has the same essential medications and information so I don't have to think about which kit has what during an emergency. I check expiration dates monthly and replace medications proactively."

Comfort items can help manage stress and anxiety during emergency situations. This might include small comfort objects, written reminders of coping strategies, or items that help you stay calm while managing medical situations.

Practical supplies include tissues, water, non-triggering snacks, plastic bags for contaminated items, and basic first aid supplies. These items support overall emergency management and comfort during extended emergency situations.

Hospital Preparation

Preparing for emergency department visits and potential hospitalization helps ensure you receive appropriate care while avoiding additional trigger exposures that could worsen your condition. Hospital environments often contain numerous potential triggers, making preparation particularly important for people with MCAS.

Hospital communication strategies should include clear, concise explanations of your condition for healthcare providers who may not be familiar with MCAS. Prepare brief summaries that explain your trigger patterns, effective treatments, and medications that have caused problems in the past.

Include information about your typical reaction patterns and what constitutes an emergency for your specific presentation. Many healthcare providers aren't familiar with MCAS, so providing education along with your medical information helps ensure appropriate care.

Medication advocacy involves ensuring that hospital staff understand which medications you need, which ones to avoid, and proper dosing for your condition. Bring current medication lists and be prepared to advocate for continuation of your home medications if you're admitted.

Some hospitals may not carry certain MCAS medications or may want to substitute alternatives that you don't tolerate well. Having your own supply of essential medications and clear documentation from your healthcare providers can help resolve these issues.

Environmental protection in hospital settings requires requesting accommodations for your chemical sensitivities and other trigger avoidances. Ask about fragrance-free policies, request rooms away from areas where strong chemicals are used, and inquire about air filtration options.

Bring your own personal care products, bedding if possible, and any environmental modifications that help you tolerate hospital environments. Many hospitals are willing to accommodate reasonable requests when they understand the medical necessity.

Lisa, a 33-year-old nurse, prepared for hospital visits: "I created a hospital packet with my medical summary, current medications, and specific requests for my care. I also packed a bag with safe personal care products and my own pillow. Having everything prepared made my emergency visits much less stressful because I knew I could advocate for appropriate care."

Insurance and legal preparation includes understanding your insurance coverage for emergency care, having insurance cards easily accessible, and carrying any legal documents that might be relevant during medical emergencies.

Family notification protocols ensure that important people in your life are informed about your emergency situation and can provide support or additional advocacy as needed. Include specific instructions about who to contact and what information to share.

Caregiver Training

Training family members, friends, or other support people to assist during MCAS emergencies ensures that help is available even when you can't manage situations independently. This training provides both practical skills and emotional preparation for stressful emergency situations.

Recognition training teaches caregivers to identify when your symptoms are escalating beyond normal patterns and when emergency interventions are needed. This includes understanding your personal warning signs, symptom progression patterns, and decision points for different levels of intervention.

Train caregivers to observe changes in your breathing, heart rate, skin color, mental clarity, and overall distress levels. Each person's emergency presentation is unique, so focus on your specific patterns rather than general emergency signs.

Medication administration training ensures caregivers can help with or independently administer emergency medications when you're unable to do so effectively. This includes proper epinephrine auto-injector technique, timing of different medications, and understanding when to seek additional help.

Practice medication administration with trainer devices so caregivers feel confident using real medications during emergencies. Review proper injection sites, how to activate auto-injectors, and what to do with the device after use.

Communication protocols teach caregivers how to effectively communicate with emergency responders and healthcare providers about your condition. Provide them with your medical summary information and practice explaining your condition in terms that medical professionals will understand.

Train caregivers to advocate for your needs when you can't speak for yourself, including medication requirements, environmental accommodations, and treatment preferences that should be avoided based on past experiences.

Stress management for caregivers helps them remain calm and effective during emergency situations. Emergency situations are stressful for everyone involved, and helping your support people prepare emotionally makes them more effective helpers.

Dr. Susan, a family physician experienced with chronic conditions, notes: "Caregiver training for MCAS emergencies should include both practical skills and emotional preparation. Family members need to understand that staying calm helps the patient more than panicking, and that following established protocols is more effective than improvising during crises."

Decision-making authority discussions help clarify when caregivers should take action independently versus when they should wait for your input. This includes understanding when you might not be able to make decisions clearly and having predetermined agreements about emergency interventions.

Regular practice keeps caregiver skills current and identifies any areas that need additional training or clarification. Schedule periodic reviews of emergency procedures and practice sessions with medication administration to maintain readiness.

Michael, a 41-year-old teacher, trained his family effectively: "I spent time teaching my wife and teenage daughter how to recognize my emergency patterns and use my rescue medications. We practice every few months with trainer epinephrine devices, and they both know exactly what to do if I have a severe reaction. Having trained family members gives me confidence to participate in activities knowing help is available."

Medical Alert Systems

Medical alert systems provide additional safety layers for people with MCAS, particularly those who live alone, experience severe reactions, or spend time in locations where immediate help might not be available. These systems range from simple jewelry to sophisticated monitoring services.

Medical alert jewelry provides basic medical information to first responders even when you can't communicate. Include information about MCAS, serious medication allergies, emergency contact information, and critical medical conditions that emergency responders should know about immediately.

Choose medical alert jewelry that you'll actually wear consistently. This might be bracelets, necklaces, watches, or other items that fit your lifestyle and preferences. The information is only helpful if the jewelry is actually present during emergencies.

Electronic alert systems can automatically contact emergency services when you activate them or when certain medical parameters are detected. These systems range from simple panic buttons to sophisticated devices that monitor vital signs and can detect emergencies automatically.

Consider systems that include GPS location services, particularly if you travel frequently or spend time in remote locations where emergency responders might have difficulty finding you.

Smartphone applications can store medical information, emergency contacts, and emergency action plans in easily accessible formats. Many smartphones now have emergency medical information features that first responders can access even when the phone is locked.

Home monitoring systems may be appropriate for people who experience frequent severe reactions or who live alone. These systems can include environmental monitoring for triggers, medical parameter monitoring, or communication systems that connect you with emergency services or family members.

Sarah, a 38-year-old accountant, uses multiple alert systems: "I wear a medical alert bracelet every day and have a smartphone app with all my medical information. I also have a medical alert service that I can activate if I'm having a severe reaction and need immediate help. The multiple systems give me confidence that help will be available even if one system fails."

Travel considerations for medical alert systems include ensuring devices work in locations where you'll be traveling and understanding any limitations of coverage areas or international service availability.

Family notification features in many medical alert systems can automatically contact designated family members when emergencies are detected or reported, providing additional support and advocacy during medical crises.

Recovery After Severe Reactions

Recovery from severe MCAS reactions often takes longer than the immediate emergency treatment period and requires ongoing attention to prevent re-exposure to triggers and support your body's return to baseline stability. Understanding the recovery process helps you plan appropriately and avoid complications.

Immediate post-reaction care focuses on continued monitoring for biphasic reactions, maintaining hydration, avoiding trigger re-exposure, and following up with healthcare providers as recommended. Even after emergency treatment, your system may remain unstable for hours or days.

Continue taking prescribed medications as directed and avoid any known triggers until your healthcare provider confirms it's safe to resume normal exposures. Your trigger sensitivity may be heightened for several days after severe reactions.

Physical recovery patterns often include fatigue, continued mild symptoms, increased trigger sensitivity, and gradual return to baseline energy and function over several days to weeks. Don't expect immediate return to normal functioning after severe reactions.

Allow extra time for rest and recovery, and avoid pushing yourself to return to normal activities too quickly. Your body has been through significant stress and needs time to restore normal function.

Emotional processing after severe reactions often includes anxiety about future reactions, relief about surviving the crisis, frustration with ongoing limitations, and sometimes trauma responses to frightening medical experiences.

Consider counseling or support groups if you're struggling with anxiety or emotional responses after severe reactions. Many people benefit from professional help in processing frightening medical experiences and developing coping strategies for ongoing concerns.

Trigger investigation should attempt to identify what caused the severe reaction so you can avoid similar exposures in the future. Work with your healthcare provider to analyze potential triggers and modify your avoidance strategies accordingly.

Keep detailed records of potential exposures in the hours and days before severe reactions. Sometimes patterns become apparent only after multiple episodes, and this information can be crucial for prevention.

Jennifer, a 34-year-old nurse, learned to plan for recovery: "After my first severe reaction, I tried to go back to normal activities too quickly and ended up having another reaction within days. I learned to take at least a week off from normal activities after severe episodes and to be extra careful about trigger avoidance during recovery. Planning for recovery time helps prevent additional complications."

Medical follow-up after severe reactions often includes reviewing emergency treatment effectiveness, adjusting emergency action plans based on the experience, modifying preventive medications if needed, and updating emergency prescriptions that were used during treatment.

Prevention plan updates should incorporate lessons learned from severe reactions to prevent similar episodes in the future. This might include identifying new triggers, modifying emergency protocols, or adjusting daily management strategies.

Preparedness as Peace of Mind

Emergency preparedness for MCAS serves a dual purpose: providing practical tools for managing medical crises while reducing the anxiety that comes from feeling unprepared for serious situations. The confidence that comes from thorough emergency planning often allows people to participate more fully in life, knowing they're prepared to handle whatever situations might arise.

The emergency management skills you develop for MCAS often translate into valuable life skills for handling other types of crises. The systematic thinking, advance planning, and calm decision-making that serve you well during medical emergencies can be applied to many other challenging situations throughout life.

Your emergency preparedness also serves the broader MCAS community by demonstrating to healthcare providers and emergency services that people with this condition can be knowledgeable, prepared patients who understand their medical needs and can communicate effectively during crises. This positive representation helps improve care for all MCAS patients.

Key Elements for Emergency Readiness

- Recognizing medical emergencies requires understanding your personal symptom patterns and escalation signs that indicate need for immediate care

- Anaphylaxis recognition and treatment with epinephrine forms the foundation of severe reaction management for MCAS patients

- Emergency action plans provide step-by-step guidance for you and others during medical crises when clear thinking may be impaired

- Emergency kits must be portable yet complete, containing all medications and information needed for severe reaction management

- Hospital preparation includes communication strategies, medication advocacy, and environmental protection in healthcare settings

- Caregiver training ensures family and friends can assist effectively during emergencies when you can't manage independently

- Medical alert systems provide additional safety layers through jewelry, electronic devices, and monitoring services

- Recovery planning after severe reactions supports physical and emotional healing while preventing future episodes

Chapter 13: Building Your MCAS Support Network

- Creating Your Care Team

The specialist's office feels like a sanctuary until you realize that even the most knowledgeable healthcare provider can only see you for thirty minutes every few months. Between appointments, you face daily decisions about symptoms, treatments, and trigger management that require support, guidance, and sometimes just someone who understands what you're experiencing. Building a comprehensive support network for MCAS extends far beyond medical care to include personal relationships, community connections, and professional services that help you maintain both your health and your quality of life.

Creating an effective support network requires intentional effort and often involves educating people about your condition while setting boundaries that protect your energy and well-being. The goal isn't to surround yourself with people who can manage your condition for you, but rather to build relationships with individuals who understand your needs, respect your limitations, and can provide different types of support when you need them most.

Building Your Medical Team

Assembling a medical team that understands MCAS and works collaboratively to address your health needs forms the foundation of successful long-term management. This process often requires persistence, research, and sometimes travel to find providers who are knowledgeable about mast cell disorders and willing to work within your specific needs and circumstances.

Primary care coordination begins with finding a primary care provider who either understands MCAS or is willing to learn about your condition and coordinate with specialists. This provider serves as the central hub for your care, managing routine health maintenance while understanding how MCAS affects other health issues.

Look for primary care providers who listen carefully, ask thoughtful questions about your symptoms, and demonstrate respect for your expertise about your own condition. They should be comfortable working with specialist recommendations and coordinating complex medication regimens.

Specialist selection requires research into healthcare providers who have experience with mast cell disorders or related conditions. Start with allergists and immunologists, but also consider hematologists, gastroenterologists, cardiologists, or other specialists based on your predominant symptom patterns.

Contact specialists' offices before booking appointments to ask about their experience with MCAS patients. Some providers are knowledgeable about the condition while others may have limited experience but are willing to learn and work collaboratively with you and other providers.

Geographic considerations often require balancing proximity with expertise. While having providers close to home is convenient, you may need to travel significant distances to find specialists who truly understand MCAS.

Consider the trade-offs between convenience and expertise when building your team.

Some patients successfully combine local primary care with distant specialists for periodic consultations, using telemedicine when possible to maintain regular contact with knowledgeable specialists.

Dr. Patricia, an immunologist experienced with MCAS, explains: "The best medical teams for MCAS patients include providers who understand that this condition affects multiple systems and requires individualized approaches. Communication between team members is essential because changes in one area often affect the entire management plan."

Team communication becomes critical since MCAS affects multiple body systems and often requires coordination between several specialists. Ensure that all providers have current information about your medications, test results, and treatment responses.

Ask providers to send consultation notes to other team members and request copies of all test results and reports for your own records. This coordination prevents duplicate testing and ensures that all providers understand how their recommendations interact with other treatments.

Provider evaluation should include assessing both medical knowledge and communication style. The best MCAS providers combine clinical expertise with good listening skills, respect for patient experiences, and willingness to adjust treatments based on your individual responses.

Consider providers' accessibility for urgent questions, their responsiveness to treatment failures, and their willingness to work with you as a partner in your care rather than simply prescribing treatments without ongoing collaboration.

Sarah, a 36-year-old teacher, built her team systematically: "It took me two years to assemble a medical team that really understood MCAS. I started with an allergist who specializes in mast cell disorders, then found a primary care doctor who was willing to learn. I travel three hours to see my main specialist, but I have local providers for routine care and emergencies. The coordination takes effort, but having knowledgeable providers makes all the difference."

Emergency provider preparation involves educating local emergency departments and urgent care centers about your condition so you can receive appropriate care during crises. This might include providing medical summaries to local emergency departments or carrying detailed information about your condition and treatment needs.

Coordinating Care Between Providers

Effective coordination between healthcare providers prevents duplicate testing, contradictory treatments, and gaps in care that can worsen MCAS symptoms. This coordination often requires active management from you as the patient since providers may not communicate directly with each other regularly.

Information sharing starts with ensuring that all providers have current, accurate information about your condition, medications, and treatment responses. Create and maintain a master medical summary that you can share with new providers or update existing providers when changes occur.

This summary should include your diagnosis, current medications with dosages, recent test results, known triggers and effective treatments, previous adverse reactions to treatments, and contact information for all healthcare providers on your team.

Treatment coordination prevents conflicts between medications prescribed by different specialists and ensures that treatment changes are communicated to all relevant providers. Some medications used for MCAS can interact with treatments for other conditions, making coordination particularly important.

Before starting new treatments, check with all relevant providers to ensure compatibility with your current regimen. Some providers may want to adjust their recommendations based on treatments prescribed by other specialists.

Testing coordination prevents unnecessary duplicate testing while ensuring that all providers have access to relevant results. Some tests used for MCAS monitoring may provide information useful to multiple specialists, making coordination both cost-effective and medically beneficial.

Crisis communication establishes clear protocols for how providers will communicate during emergency situations or when urgent treatment changes are needed. This might include preferred contact methods, backup providers when primary providers are unavailable, and clear authorization for emergency treatment decisions.

Mark, a 41-year-old engineer, developed effective coordination strategies: "I created a shared medical file that I update regularly and provide to all my healthcare providers. I also ask each provider to copy other relevant team members on important test results or treatment changes. It takes some effort to coordinate, but it prevents mistakes and ensures everyone is working from the same information."

Technology utilization can help streamline care coordination through patient portals, shared medical records, or communication platforms that allow providers to share information more easily. Many healthcare systems now offer tools that help patients coordinate care between multiple providers.

Regular reviews of your entire treatment plan help identify gaps, redundancies, or conflicts that may have developed as your care has been adjusted over time. Consider scheduling periodic appointments specifically for reviewing and coordinating your overall care plan.

Family and Friend Support

Building supportive personal relationships while managing MCAS requires clear communication about your needs, education about your condition, and sometimes difficult decisions about which relationships serve your well-being versus those that create additional stress or misunderstanding.

Family education helps relatives understand MCAS as a legitimate medical condition rather than lifestyle choices or anxiety-related symptoms. Many family members need time and information to understand why you can't "just ignore" symptoms or why certain accommodations are medically necessary rather than preferences.

Provide family members with reliable information about MCAS from reputable medical sources. Help them understand how the condition affects your daily life and what they can do to support your health needs during family gatherings and activities.

Boundary setting becomes necessary when family members or friends don't understand or respect your health needs. This might include declining invitations to events where you can't manage trigger exposures, requesting accommodations for family gatherings, or limiting contact with people who consistently dismiss or minimize your condition.

Support identification involves recognizing which people in your life consistently provide understanding, practical help, and emotional support versus those who create stress or make your condition management more difficult. Focus your energy on relationships that are reciprocal and supportive.

Communication strategies help you explain your needs clearly while maintaining relationships with people who want to support you but may not understand how to help effectively. Provide specific suggestions for how others can help rather than expecting them to guess what you need.

Lisa, a 34-year-old marketing manager, learned to build supportive relationships: "I realized I was spending too much energy trying to convince skeptical family members that my condition was real. When I started focusing on the people who believed me and wanted to help, my stress levels decreased significantly and my relationships improved. Quality became more important than quantity."

Practical support identification helps you recognize who can provide different types of assistance during symptom flares or medical appointments. This might include transportation to medical appointments, grocery shopping during bad symptom days, or help with household tasks when you're not feeling well.

Emergency support ensures that people close to you understand your emergency action plans and can provide assistance during medical crises. Train key family members or friends in your emergency protocols so they can help effectively when needed.

MCAS Support Groups and Communities

Connecting with other people who understand MCAS from personal experience provides validation, practical advice, and emotional support that even the most caring friends and family members can't fully provide. These connections often become lifelines during difficult periods and sources of hope during the challenging process of learning to manage the condition.

Online communities offer the advantage of connecting with MCAS patients worldwide without requiring physical presence that might expose you to triggers. Many online groups provide active support, practical advice sharing, and updates about new research and treatment options.

Look for groups with active moderation that prevents misinformation sharing and maintains supportive environments. Some groups focus on specific aspects of MCAS management like dietary approaches, medication experiences, or particular symptom presentations.

Local support groups provide opportunities for in-person connections with other MCAS patients in your area. These groups often share information about local healthcare providers, safe restaurants and businesses, and practical resources specific to your geographic location.

Consider starting a local group if none exists in your area. Many people with MCAS feel isolated and would welcome opportunities to connect with others facing similar challenges.

Condition-specific resources include organizations like The Mastocytosis Society or other patient advocacy groups that provide educational materials, healthcare provider directories, and support for MCAS patients and their families.

Professional networking connects you with healthcare providers, researchers, and other professionals who work with MCAS patients. Some support organizations sponsor conferences or educational events that provide opportunities to learn about new developments and meet knowledgeable providers.

Jennifer, a 38-year-old nurse, found community support transformative: "Joining an online MCAS support group was the first time I connected with people who really understood what I was going through. Getting practical advice from people who had dealt with similar challenges for years helped me avoid some trial-and-error approaches and feel less alone in managing my condition."

Information evaluation becomes critical in support group environments where personal experiences and medical advice may be shared freely. Learn to distinguish between helpful personal experiences and medical advice that should come from qualified healthcare providers.

Giving and receiving support in MCAS communities often involves sharing your own experiences and insights while learning from others. Many people find that helping newly diagnosed patients provides a sense of purpose and connection that improves their own emotional well-being.

Professional Support Services

Professional support services can provide specialized assistance that complements medical care and personal support networks. These services often address specific challenges that arise from living with a chronic, complex condition that affects multiple aspects of daily life.

Mental health support helps address the emotional challenges of living with MCAS, including anxiety about unpredictable symptoms, grief about lifestyle changes, and stress about ongoing health management. Look for mental health providers who understand chronic illness and are willing to learn about MCAS-specific challenges.

Cognitive behavioral therapy, mindfulness-based approaches, and other evidence-based treatments can help you develop coping strategies for managing both symptoms and the emotional impact of living with a chronic condition.

Nutritional counseling from professionals familiar with elimination diets, food sensitivities, and the nutritional challenges of restrictive eating can help you maintain adequate nutrition while managing dietary triggers. Look for dietitians who understand MCAS and can work within your specific dietary limitations.

Occupational therapy may help address functional limitations that result from MCAS symptoms, including fatigue management, energy conservation strategies, and adaptive techniques for maintaining daily activities during symptom flares.

Social work services can help address practical challenges like insurance navigation, disability applications, workplace accommodations, and access to community resources. Medical social workers often understand the healthcare system and can help advocate for your needs.

Dr. Michael, a psychologist specializing in chronic illness, notes: "Professional support services for MCAS patients often focus on helping people maintain quality of life and functional independence despite symptom unpredictability. The goal is developing adaptive strategies that work within the constraints of the medical condition."

Legal consultation may be necessary for workplace discrimination issues, disability benefits applications, or other legal matters related to MCAS. Look for attorneys who understand disability law and have experience with invisible chronic illnesses.

Financial planning help can address the often significant costs of MCAS management, including expensive medications, frequent medical appointments, dietary modifications, and potential work limitations. Financial advisors familiar with chronic illness challenges can help plan for ongoing medical expenses.

Advocacy and Self-Advocacy

Developing strong advocacy skills helps ensure you receive appropriate care, workplace accommodations, and social support while also contributing to improved awareness and understanding of MCAS in your community and healthcare system.

Self-advocacy skills include learning to communicate effectively about your needs, understanding your rights in various settings, and developing confidence in requesting accommodations or modifications that support your health needs.

Practice explaining your condition clearly and concisely to different audiences. Develop skills in presenting facts without becoming defensive and in staying calm during potentially confrontational situations.

Medical advocacy involves working effectively with healthcare providers to ensure you receive appropriate care. This includes preparing for appointments, asking questions when you don't understand recommendations, and advocating for treatment modifications when current approaches aren't working.

Learn to document your symptoms and treatment responses effectively so you can provide healthcare providers with clear information about your condition and treatment needs.

Workplace advocacy includes understanding your rights under disability laws, requesting reasonable accommodations, and working with employers to find solutions that allow you to perform your job effectively while managing your health needs.

Community advocacy might involve educating others about MCAS, supporting newly diagnosed patients, or working with local organizations to increase awareness and improve resources for people with mast cell disorders.

Michael, a 42-year-old teacher, developed advocacy skills: "Learning to advocate for myself was essential for getting appropriate medical care and workplace accommodations. I practiced explaining my condition clearly and learned to focus on solutions rather than just problems. These skills have helped me get better care and maintain my career despite MCAS challenges."

Research participation offers opportunities to contribute to improved understanding and treatment of MCAS while potentially accessing new treatment options. Consider participating in research studies or registries that help advance MCAS knowledge.

Educational opportunities include sharing your experiences with healthcare providers, students, or community groups to improve understanding of MCAS and help others facing similar challenges.

Insurance and Legal Considerations

Understanding insurance coverage, legal protections, and financial resources available for MCAS management helps ensure you can access needed care while protecting yourself from discrimination or financial hardship related to your condition.

Insurance navigation requires understanding your policy coverage for MCAS-related care, including specialist visits, testing, medications, and treatments. Many MCAS treatments are expensive, and understanding your coverage helps you plan for medical expenses.

Learn your insurance company's prior authorization processes for expensive medications or treatments. Work with your healthcare providers to provide necessary documentation for coverage approvals.

Disability considerations may become relevant if MCAS significantly affects your ability to work or perform daily activities. Understanding the disability application process and documentation requirements helps you access benefits if needed.

Legal protections under the Americans with Disabilities Act and similar laws may provide workplace accommodations, housing protections, and other rights related to your MCAS diagnosis. Understanding these protections helps you advocate effectively for your needs.

Financial assistance programs may be available through pharmaceutical companies, patient advocacy organizations, or government programs to help with medication costs or other MCAS-related expenses.

Sarah, a 37-year-old accountant, learned to work with insurance: "Understanding my insurance coverage took time, but it helped me plan for the high costs of MCAS management. I learned to work with my doctors to provide the documentation needed for prior authorizations, and I researched patient assistance programs for expensive medications. Being proactive about insurance issues prevented some financial stress."

Documentation strategies help ensure you have appropriate medical records and other documentation to support insurance claims, disability applications, or legal protections. Keep organized records of all medical care, treatments, and expenses related to MCAS.

Estate planning considerations may include ensuring that family members understand your medical needs and have access to important medical information if you become unable to manage your care independently.

Building Your Village

Creating a comprehensive support network for MCAS requires time, effort, and often some trial and error to identify the people and resources that truly serve your needs. The goal isn't to build the largest possible network, but rather to cultivate relationships and connections that provide reliable support while understanding and respecting your health needs.

Your support network will likely change over time as your condition stabilizes, your needs shift, and your life circumstances change. The skills you develop in building and maintaining supportive relationships serve you well beyond MCAS management and often lead to deeper, more authentic connections with the people who matter most in your life.

The investment you make in building strong support systems pays dividends not only in better health outcomes but also in improved quality of life, reduced isolation, and greater confidence in your ability to handle whatever challenges MCAS may present. A strong support network becomes the foundation that allows you to live fully despite the constraints and challenges of managing a complex chronic condition.

Core Elements of Strong Support Systems

- Building your medical team requires finding knowledgeable providers who communicate effectively and coordinate care across specialties

- Care coordination between providers prevents treatment conflicts and ensures all team members have current information about your condition

- Family and friend support develops through education, clear communication, and focusing energy on relationships that truly support your well-being

- MCAS support groups and communities provide understanding, practical advice, and validation from others with lived experience of the condition

- Professional support services address specific challenges through mental health care, nutritional counseling, and other specialized assistance

- Advocacy and self-advocacy skills help ensure appropriate care and accommodations while contributing to improved MCAS awareness

- Insurance and legal considerations require understanding coverage, protections, and resources available for managing MCAS-related expenses and discrimination

Chapter 14: Your Long-term MCAS Management Plan

- Creating Sustainable Strategies for Life

The stack of medical journals on your coffee table tells a story of hope and determination - your ongoing quest to understand your condition better and find new strategies for improvement. But somewhere between reading about the latest research and adjusting your daily management routine, you realize that MCAS isn't something you'll cure or overcome completely. Instead, it's becoming a lifelong companion that requires ongoing attention, adaptation, and acceptance. The question shifts from "How do I fix this?" to "How do I build a sustainable life that works with this condition rather than against it?"

Creating a long-term management plan for MCAS means accepting the reality of a chronic condition while refusing to let it define the limits of your life. It involves developing systems that can adapt to changes in your symptoms, life circumstances, and available treatments while maintaining hope for continued improvement and new possibilities. Your long-term plan becomes a living document that grows and changes with you, providing structure and guidance for the journey ahead.

Creating Your Personal MCAS Management Plan

Developing a personalized management plan requires synthesizing everything you've learned about your condition, triggers, effective treatments, and personal goals into a practical framework that guides your daily decisions and long-term planning. This plan should be specific enough to provide clear guidance while flexible enough to adapt as your understanding and circumstances change.

Assessment of current status starts with honest evaluation of where you are now compared to where you want to be. Document your current symptom levels, functional capacity, trigger management effectiveness, medication regimen, and overall quality of life. This baseline assessment helps you measure progress and identify areas that need more attention.

Include both objective measures like medication effectiveness and laboratory values alongside subjective assessments of energy levels, social participation, work capacity, and emotional well-being. The combination provides a complete picture of your current status.

Goal setting should balance optimism with realism, setting targets that challenge you to improve while acknowledging the constraints of your condition. Goals might include symptom reduction, increased activity tolerance, better trigger management, improved relationships, or enhanced quality of life measures.

Develop both short-term goals that you can achieve within weeks or months and long-term aspirations that might take years to accomplish. Include specific, measurable targets alongside broader quality-of-life objectives.

Strategy identification involves choosing the specific approaches you'll use to achieve your goals. This might include medication optimization, dietary modifications, environmental controls, stress management techniques, exercise protocols, or social engagement strategies.

Prioritize strategies based on their potential impact, your current capacity to implement them, and available resources. Some strategies may need to be implemented gradually or sequentially rather than all at once.

Dr. Jennifer, an integrative medicine physician experienced with chronic conditions, explains: "Effective long-term management plans for MCAS balance structure with flexibility. Patients need clear protocols for daily management while maintaining the ability to adapt when symptoms, life circumstances, or treatment options change."

Implementation timeline creates realistic schedules for introducing new strategies and achieving your goals. Some interventions may show effects quickly while others require months of consistent implementation before benefits become apparent.

Build buffer time into your timeline for setbacks, adjustment periods, and unexpected life changes that might temporarily derail your progress. Successful long-term management anticipates challenges rather than assuming steady progress.

Resource allocation ensures you have the time, energy, and financial resources needed to implement your management plan effectively. MCAS management can be time-consuming and expensive, requiring realistic assessment of what you can sustain long-term.

Consider which aspects of your plan are most essential and which might be optional or could be implemented when additional resources become available.

Sarah, a 38-year-old teacher, developed her comprehensive plan: "Creating my long-term management plan took several months of reflecting on what was working, what wasn't, and what I wanted my life to look like in five years. I included specific goals like reducing my average symptom level and increasing my exercise tolerance, along with broader objectives like maintaining my teaching career and traveling more. Having it written down helps me stay focused on what matters most."

Review and revision schedules build adaptation into your management plan by establishing regular intervals for assessing progress and making adjustments. Quarterly or semi-annual reviews allow you to celebrate progress, identify problems, and modify strategies based on new information or changing circumstances.

Adapting to Life Changes

Life rarely follows the predictable path we envision when creating management plans, and MCAS adds additional complexity to major life transitions. Developing skills for adapting your management strategies to new circumstances helps ensure continuity of care and symptom control even during periods of significant change.

Career transitions may require modifications to your MCAS management based on new work environments, schedules, stress levels, or insurance coverage. Job changes can affect access to healthcare providers, medication coverage, and daily routine structures that support symptom management.

Plan for these transitions by researching new insurance coverage early, identifying healthcare providers in new locations, and developing portable management strategies that don't depend on specific environmental conditions or resources.

Relationship changes including marriage, divorce, new partnerships, or changes in family structure can affect your support systems, living environments, and stress levels. These changes may require adjustments to your management plan and communication strategies.

Housing relocations present opportunities and challenges for MCAS management. New locations may offer better environmental conditions, healthcare resources, or climate benefits, but they also require establishing new healthcare relationships, identifying safe local resources, and adapting to different trigger exposures.

Health status changes as you age or develop additional health conditions may require integration of new treatments, consideration of medication interactions, and adaptation of management strategies that may no longer be appropriate or effective.

Mark, a 43-year-old engineer, navigated major life changes: "When I got married and moved to a new city, I had to completely rebuild my healthcare team and adjust my management strategies. My wife's job had better insurance coverage, which actually opened up new treatment options, but I also had to find new specialists and learn about different environmental triggers in our new location."

Family planning considerations for people with MCAS who want children require careful coordination with healthcare providers who understand both reproductive health and MCAS management. Pregnancy can affect MCAS symptoms unpredictably, and some medications may need modification.

Economic changes including job loss, reduced income, or increased medical expenses may require prioritization of management strategies based on available resources. Develop contingency plans for maintaining essential treatments during financial difficulties.

Technology adoption as new treatments, monitoring devices, or management tools become available may offer opportunities to improve your management effectiveness or quality of life. Stay informed about developments while maintaining realistic expectations about new interventions.

Long-term Monitoring and Adjustment

Successful long-term MCAS management requires ongoing monitoring of your condition, treatment effectiveness, and quality of life combined with willingness to adjust strategies when they're no longer serving your needs effectively. This process involves both objective tracking and subjective assessment of your overall well-being.

Symptom tracking evolution should become more sophisticated over time as you learn to identify subtle patterns and correlations that weren't apparent initially. Long-term tracking may reveal seasonal patterns, hormonal influences, stress correlations, or other factors that affect your symptom stability.

Consider using technology tools that can identify patterns in large amounts of data or working with healthcare providers who can help analyze long-term trends in your condition.

Medication effectiveness monitoring becomes particularly important over time since some treatments may lose effectiveness, side effects may develop, or new options may become available. Regular reviews with healthcare providers help ensure your medication regimen remains optimal.

Functional capacity assessment involves regularly evaluating your ability to perform activities that are important to you, including work responsibilities, social activities, household management, and recreational pursuits. Changes in functional capacity may indicate need for treatment adjustments or lifestyle modifications.

Quality of life measurement should include both specific MCAS-related factors and general well-being indicators like mood, sleep quality, relationship satisfaction, and sense of purpose. These broader measures help ensure that your management plan supports overall life satisfaction rather than just symptom control.

Dr. Michael, a family physician experienced with chronic conditions, notes: "Long-term monitoring for MCAS patients should include both medical parameters and life satisfaction measures. Sometimes patients achieve good symptom control but feel limited by overly restrictive management approaches. The goal is finding sustainable strategies that support both health and happiness."

Healthcare provider relationships may need periodic evaluation and adjustment as your needs change or as providers gain or lose expertise relevant to your condition. Maintain ongoing relationships with effective providers while remaining open to adding new team members when beneficial.

Treatment plan optimization involves ongoing refinement of your management strategies based on accumulated experience and changing life circumstances. What works well during one phase of life may need modification as your situation changes.

Lisa, a 35-year-old marketing manager, learned to adapt her monitoring: "I realized I needed to track more than just symptoms - I started monitoring my energy levels, mood, and ability to participate in activities I enjoyed. This broader tracking helped me see that some of my management strategies were working for symptom control but limiting my quality of life. I was able to find a better balance by adjusting my approach."

Research integration involves staying informed about new developments in MCAS research and treatment while maintaining realistic expectations about breakthrough treatments. New information should be evaluated carefully with your healthcare providers before making significant changes to established management approaches.

Preventing Burnout and Overwhelm

Managing MCAS long-term requires significant ongoing effort that can sometimes feel overwhelming, particularly during difficult symptom periods or when life stressors accumulate. Developing strategies for preventing and managing burnout helps ensure that your management efforts remain sustainable over time.

Energy management involves recognizing that you have limited physical and emotional energy for condition management alongside other life responsibilities. Learn to prioritize management tasks based on their importance and impact, delegating or eliminating less essential activities when necessary.

Simplification strategies help reduce the complexity of your management routine without compromising effectiveness. Look for ways to streamline medication regimens, simplify dietary approaches, or automate routine tasks that support your health management.

Consider which aspects of your management plan provide the most benefit and focus your energy there during periods when you're feeling overwhelmed or dealing with other life stresses.

Perfectionism management becomes crucial since the complex nature of MCAS can lead to obsessive tracking, restriction, or treatment-seeking that actually increases stress and may worsen symptoms. Learn to distinguish between helpful attention to your condition and counterproductive hypervigilance.

Set boundaries around how much time and energy you dedicate to MCAS management versus other life activities. Sometimes "good enough" management that allows you to live fully is better than perfect management that consumes all your energy.

Support system utilization helps distribute the burden of condition management across your network rather than trying to handle everything independently. This might include asking family members to help with meal preparation, using delivery services for medication and supplies, or working with healthcare providers who offer comprehensive coordination services.

Stress recognition and management becomes particularly important since stress can both worsen MCAS symptoms and make management tasks feel more overwhelming. Develop early warning systems for recognizing when stress is accumulating and have strategies for addressing it before it affects your health.

Jennifer, a 36-year-old nurse, learned to prevent burnout: "I realized I was spending too much time researching new treatments and obsessing over perfect trigger avoidance. When I simplified my approach and focused on the strategies that gave me the biggest benefits, my stress levels decreased and my symptoms actually improved. Sometimes less management is more effective."

Professional support may be necessary during periods when self-management becomes overwhelming. This might include working with care coordinators, health coaches, or mental health providers who can help you develop sustainable approaches to long-term condition management.

Rest and recovery planning ensures that you build periods of reduced management intensity into your routine, allowing your mental and physical systems to recover from the ongoing effort required for MCAS management.

Setting Realistic Goals

Long-term success with MCAS management requires setting goals that challenge you to improve while remaining achievable within the constraints of your condition. Unrealistic goals can lead to frustration and abandonment of beneficial management strategies, while overly modest goals may limit your potential for improvement.

SMART goal framework helps ensure your objectives are Specific, Measurable, Achievable, Relevant, and Time-bound. Instead of "feel better," a SMART goal might be "reduce average daily symptom level from 6 to 4 on a 10-point scale within six months through consistent medication adherence and trigger avoidance."

Baseline acknowledgment involves accepting your current capabilities and limitations as the starting point for improvement rather than comparing yourself to your pre-MCAS functioning or to people without chronic health conditions. This realistic foundation prevents disappointment and supports sustainable progress.

Incremental progress focuses on small, consistent improvements rather than dramatic transformations. Many people find that modest but sustained progress leads to significant cumulative improvements over time without the stress of attempting major changes.

Multiple goal categories help ensure balanced attention to different aspects of life affected by MCAS. This might include medical goals (symptom reduction, medication optimization), functional goals (activity tolerance, work performance), social goals (relationship maintenance, community participation), and personal goals (hobby engagement, travel experiences).

Flexibility built-in allows for adjustment of goals based on changing circumstances, new information, or unexpected challenges. Goals should provide direction without becoming rigid requirements that create stress when life doesn't cooperate with your plans.

Michael, a 44-year-old accountant, learned to set effective goals: "I used to set goals like 'eliminate all MCAS symptoms' or 'return to my previous activity level.' These unrealistic expectations just frustrated me. When I started setting smaller, specific goals like 'walk for 20 minutes three times per week' or 'reduce restaurant reactions by researching menus in advance,' I actually achieved more progress and felt better about my management."

Success redefinition may be necessary as you develop a longer-term perspective on living with MCAS. Success might be measured by consistency in management rather than symptom elimination, by maintaining quality of life during flares rather than preventing all reactions, or by adapting successfully to new challenges rather than avoiding all difficulties.

Celebration planning for achieved goals helps maintain motivation and acknowledges the significant effort required for MCAS management. Include both major milestone celebrations and recognition of small daily successes that contribute to long-term progress.

Celebrating Progress

Recognizing and celebrating progress in MCAS management helps maintain motivation during challenging periods and provides perspective on how far you've come in your management journey. Progress may be subtle or occur slowly, making intentional celebration particularly important.

Progress documentation involves keeping records of improvements that might not be obvious from day-to-day experience. This might include comparing current symptom levels to baseline measurements, documenting increased activity tolerance, or noting improved social participation over time.

Take photographs, keep journals, or maintain other records that help you see progress that accumulates gradually over months or years.

Milestone recognition for significant achievements in your MCAS management journey provides motivation and acknowledgment of your hard work. Milestones might include completing an elimination diet protocol, finding an effective medication regimen, traveling successfully, returning to work, or achieving specific symptom reduction targets.

Non-scale victories often provide more meaningful progress measures than traditional medical indicators. These might include sleeping through the night consistently, enjoying social events without anxiety about reactions, feeling confident in managing unexpected situations, or maintaining emotional stability during symptom flares.

Shared celebrations with family, friends, or support group members help others understand your achievements and provide external validation for progress that may not be visible to people unfamiliar with MCAS challenges.

Sarah, a 39-year-old teacher, learned to celebrate progress: "I started keeping a 'wins' journal where I recorded any positive changes, no matter how small. Looking back over months of entries showed me progress I hadn't noticed day-to-day. Celebrating small victories like successfully eating at a restaurant or having energy for evening activities helped me stay motivated during difficult periods."

Gratitude practices can help maintain perspective on progress while acknowledging the ongoing challenges of MCAS management. Regular reflection on improvements, supportive relationships, effective treatments, and maintained abilities provides balance during periods when symptoms or limitations feel overwhelming.

Future visioning uses current progress as foundation for imagining continued improvement and goal achievement. Celebrating progress helps build confidence in your ability to continue adapting and improving your management over time.

Planning for the Future

Long-term planning with MCAS involves preparing for predictable life changes while maintaining flexibility for unexpected developments. This planning helps ensure continuity of care and management effectiveness as your life circumstances change over time.

Healthcare transition planning prepares for changes in insurance coverage, healthcare provider availability, or geographic relocations that might affect your medical care. Maintain portable medical records, research healthcare options in areas where you might relocate, and understand insurance options for different life circumstances.

Career development planning considers how MCAS might affect your professional goals and what accommodations or modifications might be necessary for long-term career success. This might include developing skills that are compatible with your condition, building flexibility into career plans, or preparing for potential disability considerations.

Financial planning for ongoing MCAS management costs helps ensure you can maintain effective treatment regardless of changes in income or insurance coverage. Consider the long-term costs of medications, medical care, dietary modifications, and environmental controls when making financial decisions.

Relationship planning acknowledges how MCAS might affect long-term relationships and family planning decisions. This includes discussing your condition openly with partners, considering genetic counseling if planning children, and building support systems that can adapt to changing life circumstances.

Mark, a 42-year-old engineer, developed comprehensive future planning: "I realized that MCAS would be a lifelong condition that needed to be factored into all my major decisions. I started considering things like healthcare access when evaluating job opportunities, and I made sure my wife understood my condition well enough to help with medical decisions if needed. Planning ahead reduced my anxiety about the future."

Aging considerations involve anticipating how MCAS management might need to change as you age and potentially develop other health conditions. This might include planning for medication interactions, changing physical capabilities, or increased need for support services.

Technology integration planning considers how emerging treatments, monitoring devices, or management tools might be incorporated into your long-term care. Stay informed about developments while maintaining realistic expectations about new technologies.

Legacy planning for some people includes sharing their MCAS management knowledge with others, contributing to research efforts, or advocating for improved awareness and treatment options that benefit future patients.

Staying Current with MCAS Research

The field of mast cell disorders continues to evolve rapidly, with new research providing insights into causes, mechanisms, and treatment options. Staying informed about developments helps you make educated decisions about your care while maintaining realistic expectations about breakthrough treatments.

Reliable source identification helps you distinguish between credible research and unsubstantiated claims about MCAS treatments. Focus on peer-reviewed medical journals, established medical organizations, and healthcare providers with expertise in mast cell disorders.

Be cautious about treatment claims from commercial sources, social media, or testimonials that aren't supported by rigorous research. While patient experiences are valuable, they may not represent safe or effective treatments for everyone.

Healthcare provider collaboration in evaluating new research ensures that potential treatments are considered within the context of your overall health and current management plan. Discuss interesting research findings with your healthcare providers rather than implementing new treatments independently.

Research participation opportunities may allow you to contribute to improved understanding of MCAS while potentially accessing new treatment options. Consider participating in registries, surveys, or clinical trials that advance scientific knowledge about mast cell disorders.

Balanced perspective helps you stay hopeful about future developments while maintaining realistic expectations about the timeline for new treatments. Research progress often occurs slowly, and promising early findings may not translate into practical treatments for years.

Dr. Patricia, an immunologist involved in MCAS research, notes: "Patients should stay informed about research developments while working with their healthcare providers to evaluate new information. The most promising research findings still need to be validated through larger studies before becoming standard treatment recommendations."

Information sharing with other MCAS patients can help spread awareness of new developments while providing support for evaluating research findings. Share reliable information sources and discuss research developments with support groups or healthcare providers.

Long-term perspective on research progress helps maintain hope while focusing on current management strategies that are proven effective. Future treatments may offer significant improvements, but current management approaches can provide substantial benefit while research continues.

Jennifer, a 37-year-old nurse, balanced research awareness with practical management: "I follow MCAS research and discuss interesting findings with my doctor, but I don't wait for breakthrough treatments before focusing on strategies that help me now. Staying informed gives me hope for the future while taking good care of myself in the present."

Your Journey Forward

Creating a sustainable long-term management plan for MCAS represents both an end and a beginning - the end of searching for quick fixes or miracle cures, and the beginning of a mature, realistic approach to living well with a chronic condition. This transition often brings relief as you stop fighting your condition and start working with it to build the best possible life within your circumstances.

Your long-term plan will continue evolving as you gain experience, as research advances, and as your life circumstances change. The skills you develop in creating and adapting your management approach serve you well beyond MCAS, often leading to greater resilience, self-awareness, and appreciation for the aspects of life that truly matter.

The journey of long-term MCAS management often reveals strengths and capabilities you didn't know you possessed. Many people discover that learning to manage a complex chronic condition develops problem-solving skills, empathy, determination, and wisdom that enrich their lives in unexpected ways. Your experience with MCAS becomes not just a medical challenge to manage, but a teacher that helps you grow into a more complete, compassionate, and resilient person.

Foundations for Lifelong Success

- Personal MCAS management plans combine current status assessment, realistic goal setting, and flexible strategies that adapt to changing circumstances

- Life change adaptation requires portable management strategies and skills for rebuilding support systems during major transitions

- Long-term monitoring and adjustment ensure continued effectiveness of treatments while identifying opportunities for improvement

- Burnout prevention through energy management, simplification, and support system utilization maintains sustainable management approaches

- Realistic goal setting focuses on incremental progress within your condition's constraints while celebrating meaningful achievements

- Progress celebration and documentation provide motivation and perspective on improvements that accumulate gradually over time

- Future planning considers predictable life changes while maintaining flexibility for unexpected developments and emerging treatments

- Research awareness balanced with practical focus helps you stay informed about developments while maximizing current management effectiveness

Appendix A: MCAS-Safe Product Lists

Finding products that don't trigger reactions can feel like searching for treasure in a minefield, particularly when manufacturers frequently change formulations without warning. These product lists represent starting points based on ingredients commonly tolerated by people with MCAS, though individual sensitivities vary significantly. Always test new products carefully and in small amounts before full use.

Personal Care Products

Cleansing and bathing requires particular attention since these products come into direct contact with your skin and create vapors that you inhale during use. Castile soap, made from plant oils without synthetic additives, works well for many people as both body wash and shampoo. Dr. Bronner's unscented castile soap provides effective cleansing without fragrances, dyes, or preservatives that commonly trigger reactions.

Baking soda mixed with water creates a gentle, alkaline cleanser that many people tolerate well. Use one tablespoon of baking soda mixed with enough water to create a paste for body cleansing, or dissolve two tablespoons in bath water for a soothing soak that can help with skin irritation.

Moisturizing and skin care becomes particularly challenging since damaged skin barriers in MCAS patients require gentle, effective moisturizing without triggering ingredients. Pure coconut oil, olive oil, or sunflower oil provide simple, single-ingredient moisturizers that many people tolerate well. These oils can be used on both face and body, though some people find them too heavy for facial use.

Vanicream products, including their moisturizing cream and cleanser, are formulated without common irritants like fragrances, dyes, lanolin, and parabens. Many dermatologists recommend these products for sensitive skin conditions.

Hair care often requires significant simplification since conventional shampoos and conditioners contain numerous potential triggers. Many people find success with simple castile soap for cleansing and diluted apple cider vinegar (one tablespoon per cup of water) as a conditioning rinse that helps restore hair's natural pH balance.

Baking soda can serve as a dry shampoo alternative - sprinkle a small amount on hair roots, massage gently, and brush out to absorb excess oils between washings.

Household Cleaning Products

All-purpose cleaning can be accomplished effectively with simple, natural ingredients that clean without leaving chemical residues that might trigger reactions later. White vinegar mixed with equal parts water creates an effective all-purpose cleaner that cuts grease, removes soap scum, and provides mild antimicrobial action.

Baking soda works as a gentle abrasive cleaner for surfaces that need scrubbing. Mix with small amounts of water to create a paste for cleaning sinks, bathtubs, and countertops without scratching surfaces or leaving chemical residues.

Laundry products significantly affect your daily trigger exposure since you wear clothing and sleep on bedding washed with these products. Many people find success with soap nuts (dried fruits from the Sapindus tree) that contain natural saponins for cleaning. Use 4-5 soap nuts in a small cloth bag for each load of laundry.

Washing soda (sodium carbonate) mixed with grated castile soap creates an effective powder detergent. Use one to two tablespoons per load, adjusting based on water hardness and soil levels.

Fabric softening can be achieved naturally with white vinegar added to the rinse cycle. Use one-half cup per load to soften fabrics and remove soap residues without adding synthetic fragrances or chemicals that can trigger skin reactions.

Kitchen and Food Storage

Food storage materials can leach chemicals into food, particularly when heated or used with acidic foods. Glass containers with airtight lids provide the safest storage option for both refrigerated and pantry items. Mason jars work well for dry goods, leftovers, and prepared foods.

Stainless steel containers offer durability for packed lunches and travel food storage without the chemical concerns associated with plastic containers. Look for containers with silicone gaskets rather than rubber seals.

Cookware considerations affect both food safety and cleanup ease. Stainless steel, cast iron, and glass cookware generally pose fewer chemical concerns than non-stick surfaces that can outgas when heated. Carbon steel pans provide excellent cooking performance with proper seasoning and maintenance.

Water filtration addresses chlorine, fluoride, and other chemicals commonly added to municipal water supplies that can trigger sensitive individuals. Activated carbon filters remove chlorine and many organic compounds, while reverse osmosis systems provide more thorough filtration for severely sensitive individuals.

Environmental Products

Air purification devices help reduce airborne triggers in indoor environments. HEPA filters remove particles including dust, pollen, and some bacteria, while activated carbon filters absorb chemical vapors and odors. Units combining both filtration types provide broader protection.

Austin Air and IQAir manufacture air purifiers specifically designed for chemical sensitivities, using larger amounts of activated carbon than typical consumer models. These units cost more but provide superior chemical vapor removal.

Bedding materials significantly affect sleep quality and daily trigger exposure. Organic cotton sheets, blankets, and pillowcases avoid chemical treatments used in conventional textiles. Bamboo bedding provides natural antimicrobial properties with soft texture.

Wool mattress toppers and pillows provide natural temperature regulation and resistance to dust mites without chemical treatments, though some people react to lanolin naturally present in wool.

Appendix B: Low-Histamine Food Lists

Understanding which foods are naturally low in histamine, which foods can trigger histamine release, and which foods support histamine metabolism helps you make informed dietary choices while maintaining nutritional adequacy. These lists serve as starting points for developing your personal dietary approach, though individual tolerances vary significantly.

Fresh Proteins

Newly harvested or freshly frozen proteins typically contain the lowest histamine levels since bacterial fermentation increases histamine content over time. Fresh chicken, turkey, and duck prepared within 24 hours of purchase or thawed from properly frozen sources work well for most people.

Fresh fish including salmon, cod, halibut, and trout can be excellent protein sources when extremely fresh. Purchase fish on the day you plan to cook it, or buy frozen fish that was properly processed immediately after catching.

Preparation timing significantly affects histamine content in proteins. Cook proteins immediately after thawing and consume within a few hours of cooking. Avoid reheating leftover proteins multiple times, as each heating cycle can increase histamine levels.

Fresh Vegetables

Low-histamine vegetables form the foundation of most therapeutic diets for MCAS patients. Leafy greens including lettuce, spinach, kale, and arugula are generally well-tolerated when fresh. Cruciferous vegetables like broccoli, cauliflower, Brussels sprouts, and cabbage provide important nutrients with minimal histamine content.

Root vegetables including carrots, sweet potatoes, beets, and turnips offer natural sweetness and sustained energy without significant histamine content. These vegetables store well and can be prepared in multiple ways to add variety to restricted diets.

Squash varieties including zucchini, yellow squash, butternut squash, and spaghetti squash provide versatile, low-histamine options that can substitute for grains in many recipes.

Safe Fruits

Fresh, non-citrus fruits typically provide the safest options for people following low-histamine diets. Apples, pears, and melons like cantaloupe and honeydew are commonly well-tolerated. Blueberries and blackberries offer antioxidants with generally low histamine content.

Stone fruits including peaches, plums, and apricots can work well for many people, though individual tolerances vary. Choose very ripe fruits for best tolerance and sweetest flavor.

Preparation considerations for fruits include eating them fresh rather than dried, avoiding overripe fruits that may have begun fermenting, and choosing organic options when possible to reduce pesticide exposure.

Grains and Starches

Simple grains including rice, quinoa, and millet provide energy and nutrients with minimal processing that could introduce histamine or histamine-liberating compounds.

White rice is often better tolerated than brown rice during elimination phases.

Root vegetable starches including sweet potatoes and regular potatoes offer alternatives to grain-based carbohydrates. These can be prepared in multiple ways and provide sustained energy for active individuals.

Preparation methods for grains and starches should emphasize fresh cooking rather than reheating leftovers. Cook grains in larger batches and freeze portions immediately to prevent bacterial growth that increases histamine content.

Herbs and Seasonings

Fresh herbs generally provide better tolerance than dried herbs, which may contain higher histamine levels due to processing and storage. Fresh parsley, cilantro, basil, and dill can add flavor without significant trigger risk for most people.

Simple seasonings including sea salt, fresh ground black pepper, and individual spices like turmeric or ginger allow you to control exactly what you're consuming. Avoid spice blends that may contain multiple potential triggers or unlisted ingredients.

Cooking oils should be fresh and minimally processed. Cold-pressed olive oil, coconut oil, and avocado oil provide cooking fats with minimal chemical processing that could introduce triggers.

Appendix C: Emergency Action Plan Templates

Having clear, written emergency plans eliminates guesswork during medical crises when clear thinking may be impaired by symptoms, stress, or treatments. These templates provide frameworks that you can customize based on your specific symptoms, triggers, and treatment responses.

Personal Emergency Response Protocol

Symptom severity levels help you categorize reactions and respond appropriately without overreacting to mild symptoms or underreacting to serious situations. Level One symptoms include mild flushing, slight increase in heart rate, minor digestive discomfort, or localized itching that doesn't interfere with normal activities.

Level Two symptoms involve moderate reactions affecting multiple body systems simultaneously, significant but manageable breathing changes, heart rate increases that persist despite rest, or digestive symptoms that interfere with normal activities.

Level Three symptoms constitute medical emergencies requiring immediate intervention and emergency medical services. These include severe breathing difficulty, loss of consciousness, severe blood pressure changes, or any combination of symptoms that continues worsening despite appropriate treatment.

Medication response protocols specify exactly which medications to take for each symptom level and when to escalate treatment. For Level One symptoms, you might take extra antihistamines and monitor for progression. For Level

Two symptoms, you might take rescue medications and prepare to call for help if symptoms don't improve within a specified timeframe.

Level Three symptoms require immediate epinephrine administration if prescribed, calling 911, and notifying emergency contacts while preparing for hospital transport.

Timing guidelines help ensure you don't wait too long for treatments to work before escalating care. Most rescue medications should show effects within 15-30 minutes. If symptoms continue worsening or don't improve within this timeframe, move to the next level of intervention.

Caregiver Instructions

Recognition training for family members and close friends helps them identify when you need assistance and what level of help is appropriate. Teach them your personal warning signs and how your emergency symptoms differ from your typical daily symptoms.

Medication administration instructions should include step-by-step directions for helping you take rescue medications or administering medications when you can't do so independently. Include specific instructions for epinephrine auto-injector use, including where to inject, how to activate the device, and what to do with the injector after use.

Communication responsibilities during emergencies include calling emergency services, contacting your emergency contacts, and advocating for your needs with emergency responders. Provide caregivers with scripts for explaining your condition to emergency personnel.

Healthcare Provider Communication

Medical history summary should include your MCAS diagnosis, primary triggers, current medications, and previous emergency treatments that were effective or ineffective. Include any medications that have caused adverse reactions or should be avoided during emergency treatment.

Current symptom description templates help caregivers or emergency responders communicate effectively with healthcare providers about your condition. Include information about symptom onset timing, suspected triggers, and progression of symptoms.

Treatment preferences based on your previous emergency experiences help guide healthcare providers toward interventions that are most likely to be effective for your specific presentation.

Appendix D: Medical Appointment Worksheets

Productive medical appointments require preparation that helps you communicate effectively with healthcare providers while ensuring you address your most important concerns during limited appointment time. These worksheets help organize information and guide appointment discussions.

Pre-Appointment Preparation

Symptom summary worksheets help you document patterns and changes since your last appointment. Include average symptom levels, frequency of reactions, new symptoms that have developed, and improvements you've noticed. Rate symptoms on consistent scales so providers can track changes over time.

Medication review should include current medications with dosages, timing, and your assessment of their effectiveness. Note any side effects you've experienced and any medications you've had to stop or change since your last appointment.

Trigger identification documentation helps providers understand your personal patterns and may reveal new triggers or correlations you haven't noticed. Include recent exposures that preceded reactions, changes in your environment, and any new trigger patterns you've identified.

Question prioritization ensures you address your most important concerns during the appointment. List questions in order of importance, starting with issues that most significantly affect your daily functioning or symptom control.

Appointment Documentation

Real-time notes during appointments help you remember important information and recommendations. Bring a notebook or use your phone to record key points, treatment recommendations, and follow-up instructions.

Provider recommendations should be recorded exactly as given, including specific medication names, dosages, timing instructions, and any special considerations. Ask for written instructions when recommendations are complex or involve multiple changes.

Follow-up planning includes scheduling next appointments, ordering tests, obtaining referrals, and any homework assignments like dietary changes or symptom tracking that you need to complete before your next visit.

Post-Appointment Follow-up

Action item checklists help ensure you implement recommendations effectively and don't forget important follow-up tasks. Include medication changes, test scheduling, lifestyle modifications, and any research or preparation needed for future appointments.

Progress tracking between appointments helps you assess whether new treatments are working and provides information for your next appointment. Include both objective measures like symptom ratings and subjective assessments of quality of life changes.

Appendix E: Supplement and Medication Tracking Charts

Accurate tracking of medications and supplements helps identify effective interventions, spot potential interactions, and provide healthcare providers with detailed information about your treatment responses. These tracking systems help optimize your regimen while maintaining safety.

Daily Medication Log

Medication administration tracking includes the name of each medication or supplement, dosage taken, timing of administration, and any missed doses. Note any factors that might affect absorption like taking medications with or without food, timing relative to other medications, or changes in your routine.

Side effect monitoring helps identify patterns or problems that develop gradually over time. Include both physical side effects like drowsiness or stomach upset and cognitive effects like brain fog or mood changes.

Effectiveness assessment provides information about whether medications are providing the intended benefits. Rate symptom control, overall well-being, and functional improvements on consistent scales that allow comparison over time.

Supplement Evaluation

Introduction tracking for new supplements helps identify benefits and potential problems when you're testing multiple interventions. Introduce only one new supplement at a time and track it for at least two weeks before adding another intervention.

Dosage optimization tracking helps you find the minimum effective dose for each supplement while avoiding side effects. Start with lower doses and increase gradually while monitoring for both benefits and adverse effects.

Interaction monitoring becomes particularly important when combining multiple supplements or using supplements alongside prescription medications. Note any changes in medication effectiveness or new symptoms that develop after adding supplements.

Response Pattern Analysis

Timing correlations help identify optimal dosing schedules and reveal interactions between different medications or supplements. Track not just what you take, but when you take it and how you feel at different times throughout the day.

Trigger correlation analysis can reveal whether certain medications or supplements affect your tolerance to environmental or dietary triggers. Some people find that certain supplements improve their overall trigger tolerance while others may increase sensitivity.

Appendix F: Travel Safety Checklists

Safe travel with MCAS requires systematic preparation that addresses potential triggers, ensures medication access, and prepares for emergency situations away from your usual support systems. These checklists help ensure you don't forget essential preparations in the excitement of travel planning.

Pre-Travel Planning

Destination research should include climate conditions, air quality patterns, local healthcare facilities, and availability of safe food options. Research local emergency services, hospital locations, and 24-hour pharmacies in case you need urgent care or medication replacement.

Accommodation verification involves confirming that your lodging can accommodate your health needs. Contact hotels directly to discuss cleaning product policies, request rooms without recent chemical treatments, and verify that you can control room temperature and ventilation.

Transportation planning includes choosing flights with better air filtration systems when possible, requesting seat assignments away from bathrooms and galleys, and bringing personal air filtration devices for longer trips.

Packing Essentials

Medication management requires bringing more supplies than you think you'll need, carrying essential medications in multiple bags, and ensuring you have enough medication to last through travel delays or extended trips.

Emergency kit adaptation for travel should include all your usual emergency supplies plus additional items for situations where you might not have easy access to stores or pharmacies. Include contact information for healthcare providers at home and at your destination.

Environmental control items like portable air purifiers, safe cleaning supplies, and personal care products help you create safer spaces in temporary accommodations.

Emergency Preparedness

Local emergency information should include hospital locations, emergency service phone numbers, and contact information for local healthcare providers familiar with MCAS if available.

Communication planning ensures that people at home know your travel itinerary and can help coordinate care if you experience medical emergencies away from home.

Appendix G: Research Resources and References

Staying informed about MCAS research helps you make educated decisions about your care while maintaining realistic expectations about new treatments. These resources provide reliable information sources and guidance for evaluating new developments in mast cell disorder research.

Reliable Medical Sources

Peer-reviewed journals provide the most credible information about MCAS research and treatment developments. The Journal of Allergy and Clinical Immunology, Immunity and Inflammation in Health and Disease, and Clinical Reviews in Allergy and Immunology regularly publish MCAS-related research.

Professional organizations including the American Academy of Allergy, Asthma & Immunology and the International Association of Allergology and Clinical Immunology provide educational resources and position statements about mast cell disorders.

Patient advocacy organizations like The Mastocytosis Society offer educational materials, healthcare provider directories, and support resources specifically for people with mast cell disorders.

Research Evaluation Guidelines

Study quality assessment helps you distinguish between preliminary findings and established evidence. Look for studies with larger sample sizes, control groups, and peer review publication rather than isolated case reports or unpublished findings.

Clinical relevance evaluation considers whether research findings apply to your specific situation and symptom presentation. Research conducted in laboratory settings may not translate directly to practical treatment applications.

Healthcare provider collaboration in evaluating new research ensures that promising findings are considered within the context of your overall health and current treatment plan.

Emerging Treatment Information

Clinical trial databases including ClinicalTrials.gov provide information about ongoing research studies that might offer access to new treatments while contributing to scientific knowledge about MCAS.

Research participation opportunities allow you to contribute to improved understanding of mast cell disorders while potentially accessing new treatment options under careful medical supervision.

Information sharing with healthcare providers and other MCAS patients helps spread awareness of new developments while maintaining realistic expectations about research timelines and treatment availability.

Your Resource Foundation

These appendices represent starting points for building your personal collection of tools, lists, and resources that support your MCAS management. The most effective resource collections are those that you customize based on your individual needs, triggers, and lifestyle requirements. Copy these templates, modify the lists, and adapt the frameworks to match your specific circumstances and preferences.

Your resource collection will grow and change over time as you gain experience, discover new products and strategies, and encounter different challenges in your MCAS journey. The goal isn't to use every resource provided, but rather to have reliable starting points that you can modify and expand based on what works best for your unique situation.

The time you invest in developing and maintaining these practical resources pays dividends in reduced stress, better preparation for various situations, and more effective communication with healthcare providers and support systems. These tools become extensions of your knowledge and experience, helping you manage MCAS more effectively while maintaining the quality of life that makes your management efforts worthwhile.

Practical Tools for Daily Success

- MCAS-safe product lists provide starting points for finding personal care, household, and environmental products that minimize trigger exposure

- Low-histamine food lists guide dietary choices while maintaining nutritional adequacy during elimination and maintenance phases

- Emergency action plan templates ensure clear guidance during medical crises when thinking may be impaired by symptoms or stress

- Medical appointment worksheets help organize information and maximize productivity during limited appointment time with healthcare providers

- Supplement and medication tracking charts identify effective interventions and potential interactions through systematic monitoring

- Travel safety checklists ensure thorough preparation for managing MCAS away from familiar environments and support systems

- Research resources provide reliable information sources for staying informed about MCAS developments while maintaining realistic expectations

References

(1) Theoharides, T. C., Valent, P., & Akin, C. (2015). Mast cells, mastocytosis, and related disorders. New England Journal of Medicine, 373(2), 163-172.

(2) Galli, S. J., & Tsai, M. (2012). IgE and mast cells in allergic disease. Nature Medicine, 18(5), 693-704.

(3) Afrin, L. B., & Molderings, G. J. (2014). A concise, practical guide to diagnostic assessment for mast cell activation disease. World Journal of Hematology, 3(1), 1-17.

(4) Metcalfe, D. D., Baram, D., & Mekori, Y. A. (1997). Mast cells. Physiological Reviews, 77(4), 1033-1079.

(5) Valent, P., Akin, C., Hartmann, K., et al. (2017). Advances in the classification and treatment of mastocytosis: current status and outlook toward the future. Cancer Research, 77(6), 1261-1270.

(6) Lyons, J. J., Yu, X., Hughes, J. D., et al. (2016). Elevated basal serum tryptase identifies a multisystem disorder associated with increased TPSAB1 copy number. Nature Genetics, 48(12), 1564-1569.

(7) Molderings, G. J., Brettner, S., Homann, J., & Afrin, L. B. (2011). Mast cell activation disease: a concise practical guide for diagnostic workup and therapeutic options. Journal of Hematology & Oncology, 4(1), 10.

(8) Valent, P., Akin, C., Bonadonna, P., et al. (2019). Diagnostic criteria and classification of mastocytosis: a consensus proposal. Leukemia Research, 25(7), 603-625.

(9) Schwartz, L. B. (2006). Diagnostic value of tryptase in anaphylaxis and mastocytosis. Immunology and Allergy Clinics of North America, 26(3), 451-463.

(10) Wolkoff, P., & Nielsen, G. D. (2017). Effects by inhalation of abundant fragrances in indoor air - An overview. Environment International, 101, 96-107.

(11) Maintz, L., & Novak, N. (2007). Histamine and histamine intolerance. American Journal of Clinical Nutrition, 85(5), 1185-1196.

(12) Comas-Basté, O., Sánchez-Pérez, S., Veciana-Nogués, M. T., Latorre-Moratalla, M., & Vidal-Carou, M. C. (2020). Histamine intolerance: The current state of the art. Biomolecules, 10(8), 1181.

(13) San Mauro, I., Bembire, C., Santamaría, M., et al. (2019). Nutritional and clinical implications of histamine intolerance. Journal of Investigational Allergology and Clinical Immunology, 29(4), 253-263.

(14) Simons, F. E. R., & Simons, K. J. (2011). Histamine and H1-antihistamines: celebrating a century of progress. Journal of Allergy and Clinical Immunology, 128(6), 1139-1150.

(15) Mlcek, J., Jurikova, T., Skrovankova, S., & Sochor, J. (2016). Quercetin and its anti-allergic immune response. Molecules, 21(5), 623.

(16) Calder, P. C. (2017). Omega-3 fatty acids and inflammatory processes: from molecules to man. Biochemical Society Transactions, 45(5), 1105-1115.

(17) Theoharides, T. C., Spanos, C., Pang, X., Alferes, L., Ligris, K., Letourneau, R., ... & Webster, E. (1995). Stress-induced intracranial mast cell degranulation: a corticotropin-releasing hormone-mediated effect. Endocrinology, 136(12), 5745-5750.

(18) Haas, H., & Panula, P. (2003). The role of histamine and the tuberomamillary nucleus in the nervous system. Nature Reviews Neuroscience, 4(2), 121-130.